51885460

Qualitative research in practice

Stories from the field

Yvonne Darlington and Dorothy Scott

OPEN UNIVERSITY PRESS
Buckingham • Philadelphia

For our fathers

Bernard Olsson Darlington
and
Arthur Henry Scott

Open University Press
Celtic Court
23 Ballmour
Buckingham
MK IH IXW
Email: enquiries@openup.co.uk
world wide web: www.openup.co.uk
and
325 Chestnut Street
Philadelphia, PA 19106, USA

First published in 2002
by Allen & Unwin, Australia

A catalogue record of this book is available from the British Library.

ISBN 0335 21147 X

Typeset by Midland Typesetters
Printed by South Wind Productions, Singapore

10 9 8 7 6 5 4 3 2 1

Contents

Contents

Contents

The researchers

Tim Booth is Professor of Social Policy at the University of Sheffield. He graduated in Sociology from the University of Essex and, after a spell as a research officer in a social services department, joined the University of Sheffield in 1975. His current research interests are parenting by people with learning difficulties, advocacy and supported parenting, narrative research with inarticulate informants and the uses of fictional methods in social research. He has published four books and numerous journal articles in the area of parents with learning difficulties. Much of his work in this area has been conducted jointly with Wendy Booth.

Wendy Booth is a Research Fellow in the Department of Sociological Studies at the University of Sheffield. Wendy is involved in the field of parents with learning difficulties, as a researcher and an advocate. She has, with Tim Booth, published four books and numerous journal articles on their research with parents with learning difficulties and the children of parents with learning difficulties. She has also completed an action research project which provided advocacy support for parents with learning difficulties and is involved in a further project which offers supported learning opportunities to mothers with learning difficulties. She is the adviser to Huddersfield People First and writes a regular column in *Viewpoint*, the monthly newspaper of Mencap.

Anne Coleman began her professional social work career in 1990 as the social worker/welfare coordinator at an inner city drop-in centre for homeless people. Her work there was the start of an abiding interest in the issue of homelessness, and in understanding alternative discourses and meanings. As well as direct practice, grounded research and its links with policy processes and outcomes became central to her work. Anne completed her doctoral research on the meaning of public space to homeless people in an inner city area of Brisbane. She has been a research officer and lecturer in the School of Social Work and Social Policy at the University of Queensland and has recently taken up a position as Senior Policy Officer with the Department of Housing, Queensland. In this role, she maintains contact with homeless people in the inner city, and continues to be involved in policy and research relating to homelessness.

Yvonne Darlington lectures and researches in the School of Social Work and Social Policy at the University of Queensland. She has previously practised as a social worker in mental health and family law settings. Within the School, she teaches in the areas of child welfare, evaluation research and legal aspects of social work practice. She has completed qualitative research on adult women's experiences of having been sexually abused in childhood; worker, client and family experiences of hope in mental illness; young adults' experiences of having been the subject of contested Family Court proceedings as children; and child welfare workers' understandings of physical child abuse. She is currently involved in a project, Using Knowledge in Practice (UKIP), that is assisting child protection workers to develop skills in evidence-based practice.

Liz Kelly began researching in 1980 for her PhD on women's experience of violence. In 1987 she became the first staff member of the Child and Woman Abuse Studies Unit at the University of North London, and has worked there ever since. A feminist activist prior to becoming a researcher, she has continued to work in an unpaid capacity, either directly with women or as an activist, alongside her professional involvement in this issue. Her research interest in this area developed out of a dissatisfaction about the ways in which different forms of violence had become separated in research and in service provision, when these things are not separated in women's and children's lives, and this has been a continuing theme in her research. With her colleagues at the Unit, she has completed about twenty-two different projects, mainly on child sexual abuse, domestic violence and rape.

Catherine McDonald lectures and researches in the School of Social Work and Social Policy at the University of Queensland. Her research interests are the non-profit human services sector, the mixed economy of welfare, the reconstruction of the welfare state and shifts in the institutional arrangements supporting people. Her professional background is in social work although she identifies more broadly as a person working in and around community human services. She has worked as a social worker in child protection, residential care and psychiatric social work, in Australia and Malaysia. She is the author of thirteen journal articles and several book chapters. Most of her writing is on the non-profit sector, the mixed economy of welfare, and theorising the reconstruction of welfare. She is currently engaged in several research projects, including a large research project on the reconstruction of the community services industry.

Robyn Munford is Head of the School of Sociology, Social Policy and Social Work at Massey University, Palmerston North. She has qualifications in both social work and sociology from Massey University and the University of Calgary. She has lectured extensively at both undergraduate and postgraduate levels on community development, disability services and policy, generic social work practice, feminism and social work, and qualitative methods. She has extensive research experience in the disability and family work fields. Her research interests include women and management, disability policy, family policy and effective strategies for achieving family change, as well as issues around the creation of environments conducive to the development of child and family well-being.

Jackie Sanders is the Research Director of the Barnardos Child and Family Research Centre in New Zealand. Jackie has management experience in the for-profit and health sectors and also in the provision of welfare and early childhood services to families. She is currently involved in several research projects which have children and families as their focus. The projects include research into factors that are associated with positive change in families seeking support from a home-based family support service, and community research into factors associated with family well-being. These research programs are funded by the Public Good Science Fund—a government body which supports social science research in New Zealand.

Dorothy Scott is Associate Professor in the School of Social Work at the University of Melbourne and is currently on secondment as the Executive Director of the Ian Potter Foundation. Her academic background is in history and social work. Her practice and policy interests are in child welfare, mental health and maternal and child health. She has taught practice research at a postgraduate level in Australia and overseas, and has written seminal papers on epistemological and hermeneutic issues in social work. She has undertaken extensive qualitative research in the fields of child welfare history, maternal and child health, and child protection. Her current research interests are the history of child protection, and social support in the transition to motherhood. In 1999 she was awarded a medal of the Order of Australia for her contributions in the field of child abuse, post-partum psychiatric illness and social welfare education and research.

Caroline Thomas is a Research Fellow at Cardiff Law School, Cardiff University. She graduated in Social Policy from the University of Exeter in 1982. After working in the health service and voluntary sector, she joined Bristol University's Socio-Legal Centre for Family Studies in 1991, where she was involved in several studies to evaluate the *Children Act 1989*. Later she moved to Cardiff Law School to take the lead role in a study of older children's views and experiences of the adoption process. Caroline is currently on secondment to the UK Department of Health, managing the children's social care research program.

Cheryl Tilse is a lecturer and researcher in the School of Social Work and Social Policy at the University of Queensland. She has practised as a social worker in Australia and Canada in mental health, rehabilitation and corrective services. Within the School, she teaches in the areas of knowledge and practice, the organisational context of practice and practitioner research. Her research interests are in practitioner-based research, the organisational and policy context of practice and in ageing and aged care policy. Her current research includes evaluating housing options for older people, enhancing family and resident participation in aged care facilities, the legal aspects of later life decision-making around health care and accommodation options, asset management and the financial abuse of older people, and the implementation of user charges in aged care services. She is a member of the editorial board of the *Australasian Journal on Ageing*.

Angelina Yuen-Tsang is currently Associate Head and Associate Professor of the Department of Applied Social Sciences of the Hong Kong Polytechnic University. She obtained her BSocSc in Social Work from the University of Hong Kong in 1975, MSW from the University of Toronto in 1978, MEd from the University of Manchester in 1983, and her PhD from the University of Hong Kong in 1995. She is now the President of the Hong Kong Social Workers Association and is a board member of numerous social welfare organisations in Hong Kong. She is actively involved in the development of social work education in mainland China and in training social work educators in China. Her main research interest is on social support networks in Chinese communities using a grounded theory approach. She is conducting several research projects on social support networks of women, the elderly and the unemployed in China.

Table of research studies

Tim and Wendy Booth—*Parenting Under Pressure: Mothers and Fathers with Learning Difficulties* (1994) ('Parenting under pressure')

Anne Coleman—Five star motels: spaces, places and homelessness in Fortitude Valley (2001) ('Five star motels')

Yvonne Darlington—The experience of childhood sexual abuse: perspectives of adult women who were sexually abused in childhood (1993) ('The experience of childhood sexual abuse')

Liz Kelly—*Domestic Violence Matters* (1999)

Catherine McDonald—Institutionalised organisations? A study of non-profit human service organisations (1996) ('Institutionalised organisations?')

Robyn Munford and Jackie Sanders—*Working Successfully with Families* (1996, 1998, 1999)

Caroline Thomas—*Adopted Children Speaking* (1999)

Dorothy Scott—Child protection assessment: an ecological perspective (1995) ('Child protection assessment')

Dorothy Scott—Identification of post-partum depression by child health nurses (1987a, 1987b, 1992) ('Identification of post-partum depression')

Cheryl Tilse—The long goodbye: the experience of placing and visiting long-term partners in a nursing home (1996) ('The long goodbye')

Angelina Yuen-Tsang—*Towards a Chinese Conception of Social Support: A Study on the Social Support Networks of Chinese Working Mothers in Beijing* (1997) ('Social support networks of Chinese working mothers in Beijing')

Preface

In this book we aim to bridge the gap between theory and practice and between academic and practice contexts in qualitative research. We do this through the use of research practice narratives to illustrate stages of the research process. It is more a book about 'doing' research and 'being' a researcher than about 'how to' do research.

In Chapter 1 we begin with an exploration of the journey from practice to research—how to generate a research question and how some research questions that arise in the human services might best be explored through a qualitative research design. The ensuing chapters focus on specific stages of the research process, through data collection, analysis and writing up to, finally, the shift from research back to practice.

Chapter 2 addresses ethical issues and the organisational context of research.

Chapters 3, 4 and 5 focus particularly on data collection. In Chapter 3 we consider in-depth interviewing and in Chapter 4, observation. Chapter 5 addresses challenges involved in interviewing children and people with an intellectual disability, exploring different ways in which research can be modified to better meet the needs of these groups of participants.

In Chapter 6 we consider some approaches to mixing qualitative and quantitative methods where one method alone cannot adequately address a research question. This is a common approach in the human services, where the issues researchers are faced with are often complex and multi-faceted.

In Chapter 7 we consider some data analysis processes that are common to many approaches to qualitative research. Chapter 8 focuses on presentation and writing up, exploring different ways of writing up research so that the findings can be communicated with different audiences. Finally, in Chapter 9 we conclude with the feedback loop which takes us from research findings back to practice and policy implications—as practice research is a means to an end, not an end in itself.

The book provides an introduction to qualitative research, primarily through the medium of practice-based stories that illustrate particular stages of the research process. Each chapter includes at least two and often more 'stories from the field'. Thus the reader will not necessarily find 'the answer', but will discover how others have dealt with various aspects of qualitative research practice. This reflects our belief that there is great value in learning from others' experience. We hope the book will encourage creativity and, by showing how other researchers have dealt with particular issues, act as an aid to research troubleshooting. The book is thus also a showcase of the variety of qualitative research that is being done in different fields within the human services. By bringing these examples together, we hope to share them with a wider audience than the specific field to which each study belongs.

We have written the book for anyone with an interest in qualitative research, but particularly for students and practitioners in the human services. We hope the researcher perspectives we have presented will be of value to students and practitioner researchers alike, enabling them to draw on others' experience in the design of their own projects.

We were clear from the start that we wanted the book to include comments from researchers about how they do qualitative research. We envisaged not so much personal experiences about what it is like to be a qualitative researcher as comments about how researchers made their choices about what to do, and how the day-to-day research context interacts to shape what is possible. Through our discussions, this evolved into the idea of conducting in-depth interviews with researchers and including sections from those interviews in relevant chapters. We decided first what issues we wanted to include, and then sought out researchers who seemed to us to have grappled with at least one of those issues in an interesting or innovative way.

The work of all of the researchers included in the book was

known to us, either through personal contact or through their writing, and we chose each researcher deliberately, with a particular chapter of the book in mind. This reflected the reason we included them and focused the major part of the interview, but all the interviews were more broad-ranging than the one topic. In this way, we pre-selected the researchers to be included in the chapters on ethics and organisations, interviewing, observation, tailoring research to suit the needs of participants and mixed methods.

We decided to include excerpts from a selection of the researchers in the first and final chapters and in the chapters on data analysis and writing up, but without anyone in mind ahead of the interview. To this extent, the writing of the book has been a parallel process with qualitative research. We did not pre-empt the content areas included in these chapters. Rather, we sorted through the data (the interview transcripts) to see who had had interesting things to say on these topics—and we had plenty to choose from!

It will be obvious to any reader that we have edited the transcripts. We selected excerpts from what were very long interviews, some as long as three hours, and none less than an hour and a half. We also made the choices about where to place the excerpts. Some clearly could have fitted equally well into more than one chapter. This reflects the messiness of research! The text is also more polished than the transcripts. We have deleted repetitions and digressions and generally edited the interview text to make it flow more smoothly as written text. We struggled with this and tried to strike a balance between remaining as true as possible to the actual spoken word while maximising readability. Above all we wanted to get the message across about what the researchers were saying, and 'smoothing out' the text was important to this. We sent all of the excerpts to the researchers for comment before their final inclusion in the book, and we have made the corrections they requested. Where the researchers asked us to do more to tidy up the expression and grammar, we took this as validation of and support for the editing decisions we had made and, in some cases, permission to do more.

We know many other researchers whose work could have had a place in this book. In the end we decided to limit the overall numbers and to use multiple excerpts from the interviews. We had the data we needed and it seemed important to use what we could and not collect more that we would be unable to use. We also liked the continuity and coherence afforded by following the researchers and their studies through different stages of the research process and hope this helps the reader to become familiar with their work and to follow the threads through the book.

We thank each of the researchers we interviewed—for the readiness with which they agreed to participate in the project, and for their willingness to share their inside stories, given the many unknowns associated with where they would end up. Our thanks also go to Ann Tierney and David Tregaskis for transcribing the interviews, and to Lesley Chenoweth for her helpful comments on Chapter 5.

As writing the book came to a close, we were struck by how our own experiences and those we had drawn from our fellow researchers were becoming synthesised into a collective 'practice wisdom'. We hope that others, including those who may be inspired by reading this book, will add their own experiences of research to what we have produced. In this way, new issues and debates will arise which may challenge what we have said and so extend the emerging body of knowledge on qualitative research in the human services.

1

From practice to research

In the varied topography of professional practice, there is a high, hard
ground where practitioners can make effective use of research-based
theory and technique, and there is a swampy lowland where
situations are confusing 'messes' incapable of technical solution. The
difficulty is that the problems of the high ground, however great their
technical interest, are often relatively unimportant to clients or the
larger society while in the swamp are the problems of greatest human
concern (Schon, 1983, pp. 42–3).

The swampy lowland of practice in the human services is a place
where there are rarely control groups, where operationalising key
constructs in behavioural terms is highly problematic (Is happiness
the frequency of smiling behaviour?), where the politics of the
setting are often overwhelming and where values and ethical issues
are critical and complex. This book has more to do with the swampy
lowland than the high hard ground. However, there is a lot of territory in the human services field which connects these two parts of
the landscape and we believe that researchers in the human services
should be creating terraces which link the two parts of the terrain,
not creating territorial disputes.

The belief that 'science makes knowledge, practice uses it' has
been claimed to be one of the assumptions of positivism (Rein &
White, 1981, p. 36), yet 'scientific' methods of investigation have
great difficulty coping with the dynamic and complex social world
of the human services. Qualitative research has an important role to

play in understanding this world and in complementing other forms of knowledge.

Qualitative research methods have descended from several disciplines and belong to twenty or more diverse traditions (Miller & Crabtree, 1992). Despite such diversity the core qualitative methods can be described as follows:

- In-depth interviewing of individuals and small groups.
- Systematic observation of behaviour.
- Analysis of documentary data.

In this book we will focus on the first two methods. The techniques we will explore in relation to the analysis of transcripts of interviews or observational field notes are also applicable to pre-existing documentary data.

Qualitative research is not new. Historians have always analysed documentary evidence, much of it non-quantitative data such as correspondence, as their primary source material, and through oral history methods have added in-depth interviewing to their repertoire in recent decades. Anthropology, from its conception as a discipline in the mid-nineteenth century, used qualitative methods such as field observation and informant interviewing to understand cultural patterns and social relationships. Sociology has always drawn upon both quantitative and qualitative methods, such as in the influential Chicago school of urban research in the 1920s, and has often utilised both approaches. Organisational theory has been based largely on case studies created from an amalgam of observation, documentary material and interviews.

In recent years specialisations such as medical anthropology and medical sociology have relied heavily on qualitative methods to explore issues relating to health and illness, from the micro-context of the hospital ward or clinic through to the broader sociocultural context. Qualitative methods have extended well beyond the boundaries of the social sciences in academia. Market research was originally based on the social survey but now complements this with focus groups to tap the processes and nuances of consumer opinion, as does research on public opinion and voting intentions.

Qualitative research in the human services

For well over a decade there has also been a growing interest in qualitative research by academics within nursing, education and social work as they attempt to struggle with the issues which arise in their particular part of the swampy lowlands. Research methods such as in-depth interviewing and participant observation are particularly well suited to exploring questions in the human services which relate to the meaning of experiences and to deciphering the complexity of human behaviour.

Understanding the significance of past or current experiences lends itself to methods such as in-depth interviewing in which trust and rapport are essential if an individual is to share thoughts and feelings. Some questions lend themselves to systematic observation in order to identify the dynamics which may be operating in a particular group or organisation, or the interaction of different social groups within a community.

This book draws upon a range of qualitative studies in the human services to illustrate how researchers develop their research question, work their way through a minefield of ethical and political obstacles, systematically collect appropriate data, analyse it with rigour and then disseminate the findings and implications of the research.

The interviews we have conducted with qualitative researchers for this book have been taped and transcribed and excerpts from a few of these studies are used in each chapter in order to highlight aspects of that chapter's theme. In many ways this is itself a parallel process to qualitative research. In some chapters, including this one, we also draw upon our own qualitative studies—when we do so, we speak to the reader in the first person in order to highlight that the authorial voice is always present in qualitative research.

In this chapter we explore how the questions which arise from practice in the human services can be addressed by both quantitative and qualitative approaches and sometimes by both at the same time. We then draw upon several qualitative studies to examine how research questions can emerge from different contexts and address very different questions.

Our examples cover diverse fields and units of attention and include women who were sexually abused in childhood; parents with an intellectual disability; maternal and child health nurses' assessment of post-natal depression; a community of homeless people under siege in an inner city area; and a large service system consisting of a large number of organisations.

While most of the researchers were not working as practitioners at the time of the inception of their studies, nearly all of them bring to their research many years of experience working in the human services. Regardless of the researchers' backgrounds, all of the studies described have important implications for the way in which policies, programs and services are developed and delivered.

Generating research questions

The world of research and the world of practice have remained fairly separate. Yet every day those working in the human services field, be it with individuals, families, groups or whole communities, generate multiple questions from their practice. Some of the questions which arise are clinical hypotheses—ideas about the possible background features or presenting features in a particular individual or family, or working hypotheses about interventions that may result in a certain outcome in a particular case. Beyond the clinical level are similar questions which might relate to a whole group of service users, or how to collaborate with others to bring about a change in an organisation, a community or an entire service system.

Most practitioners would not think of such questions as research. If they had the time to write down their ideas or to share one of their questions with colleagues it might start with a phrase such as 'I wonder if . . .?' or 'I've got a hunch that . . .'. Given that research has traditionally been conceived within a 'hypothetico-deductive' model of science, it is little wonder that practitioners' questions which come from the swampy lowland do not come in the form of 'falsifiable' propositions.

The often tacit nature of clinical judgement leads the practitioner and others to dismiss their professional knowledge as unresearchable 'intuition' (Scott, 1990). This type of knowing is not always easy to state explicitly in a generalisable propositional form, leading Schon (1983) to observe that experienced professionals often know more than they can say.

Practitioners are often intimidated and alienated by the very notion of 'research'. In a word-association exercise one of us has done many times with groups of experienced health, education and welfare practitioners, words that have been offered in relation to the word 'research' include: objective, hard, cold, scientific, measurement, accurate, factual, time-consuming, difficult, prestigious, tedious, expert. When asked to offer words which sprang to mind

4

in relation to 'practice', the following were among those typically offered: subjective, people, busy, messy, difficult, soft, warm, pressured, flexible.

The researcher–practitioner split

The dichotomies between notions of objective and subjective and between art and science seem to parallel the dichotomy between the world of research and the world of practice. This dichotomy is not new and has been the focus of a debate which has unfolded over the past half century. The 'researcher–clinician split' which occurred in psychology in the 1950s has been attributed to the attack mounted by Eysenck on psychotherapy as pseudo-science (Hersen & Barlow, 1976). Yet behaviourism strongly assisted in the development of the clinician-researcher or practitioner-scientist in psychology, with single subject research designs and other quasi-experimental methods being refined for use in clinical settings.

In the 1970s extreme behaviourist positions were strongly challenged by the rise of humanistic psychology. The faith in empiricism to deliver knowledge for practice in the human services was still strong in some quarters in the 1980s. 'The issue of whether one can measure the subtleties of human nature and interaction will cease to be a problem once devised measurement rules can be shown to have a rational and empirical correspondence to reality' (Bostwick & Kyte, 1981, p. 677). Yet in the same era the emergence of emancipatory and feminist research traditions pushed the boundaries of research methods even further to address the power imbalance between the researcher and the researched and to allow the voice of the 'subject' to be heard through qualitative research.

In the 1990s the extension of 'evidence-based practice' from medicine to the rest of the health field, as well as to education and social welfare, gave empiricist approaches a new vigour in a context of resource scarcity in which effectiveness and efficiency were dominant concerns for government. Yet in the same decade the growth of post-modernist traditions in the social sciences led to a strong resurgence of interest in qualitative research and saw its expansion into fields such as discourse and narrative analysis in cultural studies.

A rapprochement of sorts is occurring between quantitative and qualitative research methods within the social sciences. In recent years we have seen the terms 'practice research' and 'practitioner-researcher' transcend the narrow behaviourist model of the clinician-scientist and draw upon a broad range of both quantitative and qualitative modes of inquiry. We do not wish to dichotomise quantitative and qualitative methods of investigation here, as the questions which arise in the human services require a broad repertoire of research approaches.

Quantitative and/or qualitative methods?

Some questions are readily transformed into testable propositions and can be investigated using quantitative methods. Sometimes this involves a major endeavour to collect and analyse the necessary data but it can also involve the analysis of data which can be collected easily or which already exists. For example, hypotheses such as 'Clients who are rung the day prior to an appointment will be more likely to keep the appointment' or 'Clients who are offered an appointment within three days of making the appointment will be more likely to keep the appointment' are easy to test even in a small human service organisation.

The client information systems and management information systems used in human service agencies today provide an extraordinary reservoir of quantitative data which can be analysed very simply to answer many questions about service user characteristics, the nature of service provision and, to some extent, the outcomes of service. Furthermore, hypotheses about patterns of presentation to a service in relation to different sections of the community can be relatively easily investigated if the demographic profile of an area is known. Thus the over- or under-representation of males or females or people of different age groups, occupational status or ethnic backgrounds can be identified. The reasons why this might be so cannot be so easily investigated using quantitative methods, however, and qualitative methods may have a place in exploring how people define their needs and why and how they seek assistance in certain places.

Similarly, feedback from those using services can be obtained easily through routine client satisfaction scales which rate different aspects of a service, but hearing how the clients have benefited or not from a service in their own words will require more than a standard quantitative approach. To tap both dimensions of consumer feedback may require a combination of questionnaire items with predetermined response categories as well as a number of open-ended questions such as 'How did you expect to benefit from this service?', 'What were the most useful/least useful aspects of the service?' and 'What suggestions could you make for improving the service?'

The latter type of question does not presuppose a particular classification of responses, and in analysing such data the researcher has to inductively derive categories from the individual responses. This involves making qualitative judgements about their meaning before they can be allocated to a particular category. Of course, one can 'allow the data to speak for itself' by reproducing all of the individual responses but this merely leaves the task of making sense of the responses up to the reader. It is possible to turn qualitative data of this nature into quantitative data if the categories are clearly defined. Thus, with some risk to the diversity and nuances of the data, and recognising that those with literacy problems may remain unheard, it is possible to take some qualitative data from the swamp up to the high hard ground and analyse it there.

In other situations, questions from both the high ground and the swampy lowland emerge from the same setting but cannot be transformed into quantitative data. Thus a social worker in an oncology unit of a hospital who is interested in establishing a support group for women with gynaecological cancers may ask herself a range of very different questions. As she looks at a list of the patients in a particular ward she may ask the following sorts of questions: How many women in the ward at this time have a similar diagnosis? How many with this diagnosis are at a similar stage in the trajectory of their condition? What is their average length of admission? These are fairly straightforward numerical questions for which the data already exist.

The next question she may ask is of a very different order: What are the multiple meanings of such a diagnosis for these women and significant others in their lives at this time? This is a hermeneutic question, that is, it is about the construction of meaning. The responses to such a question are unlikely to be easily classified into mutually exclusive categories that could be quantitatively analysed and, even if they were, it is likely that much damage would be done to their complexity and subtlety. One of us has argued that 'meaning construction' is at the heart of much of the work in the human services field and that the core traditional professional tools of client-centred interviewing and observation are not dissimilar to the qualitative research methods of in-depth interviewing and participant-observation (Scott, 1989).

The same question which our social worker asks about the meaning(s) of gynaecological cancers could equally be asked by a medical sociologist. The difference would be, however, that for the professional practitioner such a question is immediately and directly connected with what she then does and leads to a series of equally complex questions. Would it be helpful or unhelpful to form a support group for these women? What would be the best way to facilitate such a group? How could one know whether the group was successful or not? For whom might it have been helpful or unhelpful and why? How might forming such a group affect and be affected by the current pressures on staff in the ward and the inter-professional tensions and dynamics?

Researchers could explore (and some have done so) certain aspects of these questions using quantitative methods, for example, by investigating the long-term outcomes of cancer support groups in relation to years of survival. On the other hand, qualitative methods may allow some of the questions to be explored in a different way. For example, the views of the women themselves on their experience in a group and what they may have found helpful or unhelpful would be important.

Stories from the field

Here are examples of how some of the researchers we draw upon in this book generated the questions which led to their decision to adopt a qualitative approach. They illustrate something of the diversity of issues which can be explored in qualitative research and the range of methods which can be used. They also reveal the centrality of the researcher as a person to the whole process.

Tim and Wendy Booth—Parenting under pressure

This study (Booth & Booth, 1994a) is about the parenting experiences of UK parents with an intellectual disability. The study involved unstructured interviews with 33 parents, followed by more intensive work with thirteen of those parents—six couples and one single parent—over the course of a year. Wendy and Tim were interviewed together for this book. We talk with them again later about their approach to interviewing people with learning difficulties and about how they wrote up the study. Wendy is talking here about how they came to be interested in this area.

> *Wendy:* I came into it about the mid-eighties, when we were looking at the closure of the long stay hospitals . . . as a researcher I was looking at how it affected families, this change of policy; but in and amongst getting to know parents whose sons and daughters were in hospital, I also got to know some of the sons and daughters. As they came out, they moved into their home towns, and whilst I was doing that research . . . I came across a mother with learning difficulties, and at that point, neither Tim nor I had ever considered that people with learning difficulties had children. She was being helped in a special care unit after the birth of her second child . . . and that's what really got us interested. I knew some of the professionals in the area who might be able to help us and give us an idea of how many parents might be around, and talking with them, they knew seven mothers, and that's when we put in for a grant.

Anne Coleman—Five star motels

For her PhD research, Anne Coleman (2001) was interested in exploring the connection between homeless people and the public spaces they use. She situated the study in Fortitude Valley, an inner city suburb of an Australian city. The study was conducted over a period of some years at a time of urban redevelopment and conflict in the area about homeless people. It was a multi-method study, involving observation, in-depth interviews, informal interviews and document analysis. We talk with Anne again later in the book about negotiating entry to the community, using observation as a data collection method, analysing data, the readings of her work which she held for homeless people who had been involved in the study and the impact of the study. Here, Anne talks about how she became interested in doing research with homeless people.

Anne: The central research question was 'What do public spaces in that area mean to people who have been homeless there for quite some time?' So I was really interested in exploring the connection between homeless people and the public spaces they use . . . I started work with homeless people in 1990 and I'd never really had any contact with them before but the way they saw their lives and the things that happened to them made perfect sense to me . . . after three years' contact with homeless people in a drop-in centre, as well as learning an immense amount I started to form relationships with people. I suppose it was partly because their lives aren't full of a lot of significant other people, but I became important to people quickly. The other side for me was that the privilege of being able to learn things from people who lived so close to where I lived, but in a different world, really took hold of my imagination, and I became more and more interested in trying to understand how all of us as human beings share certain things in common but still make unique meanings, because of the life journey that we've been on. After I finished that three years' work as a social work practitioner I was lucky enough to be able to stay in the area. I kept in contact with people, and in doing that of course more learning took place and there was more exchange of skills and ways of looking at the world. And just as I was starting to think about doing some further study, I became aware that many of the people that I knew in the Valley who had been homeless were still using those public spaces even though there'd been this really big urban renewal process in the area. So what happened was that people were really under pressure . . . they were being moved on by the police and their gear was taken out of parks and dumped at night and all sorts of things had happened, but in spite of the obvious message that they kept getting sent—'We don't really want you here any more'—they kept going back and using these spaces. So I started to think that maybe I didn't quite understand what these spaces meant to these people, that in fact it wasn't just any public

10

space—that there was something about these specific places and these specific people and it was the connection between those two things that was important.

Yvonne Darlington—The experience of childhood sexual abuse

Yvonne talks here about the background to her study, published in 1996.

Yvonne: In the early to mid-1980s I was working as a social worker in a community mental health centre. At that time, child sexual abuse was only just emerging as a recognised area of public and professional interest— a number of articles had been printed in the press and popular magazines, and child protection responses were beginning to be developed.

There was certainly little recognition of child sexual abuse as a legitimate area for mental health intervention. Nevertheless, in my position as a female counsellor in a mental health team, many women who had sought assistance in relation to depression, feelings of worthlessness or relationship problems, disclosed childhood sexual abuse in the course of counselling. For some, the abuse had been previously disclosed, either at the time of the abuse or later, and for others this was the first time they had talked about the abuse with anyone.

Many, though not all, of the women I spoke with linked their present problems to their sexual abuse in childhood and there were also similarities in the ways they talked about what had happened and what it had meant in their lives. I became interested in the ways in which these women understood their experience of childhood sexual abuse and its long-term impact on their lives.

This was the starting point of what turned out to be a circuitous route to finally settling on a qualitative methodology for my PhD research. I experienced considerable pressure to do a quantitative study, but

11

however I constructed and reconstructed my research questions, there was always one that I returned to—how do women who have been sexually abused as children make sense of that experience? The strength of that original idea, and my concern that women's perspectives had been missing from the research in this field, won through in the end. I conducted two in-depth interviews each with ten women—one lengthy interview in which they talked about their experiences of childhood sexual abuse and the impact they felt it had had on their lives, and a shorter interview, about four to six weeks later, in which they talked about how they had experienced the first interview. The second interviews provided some useful insights about what it is like to be a research participant and I have included some of this material later in the book.

Catherine McDonald—Institutionalised organisations?

Catherine McDonald used a mixed method approach involving a survey and semi-structured interviews for this study (McDonald, 1996). Catherine talks here about how she became interested in the application of neo-institutional theory to the non-profit sector in Queensland. We talk with her again about her use of mixed methods and how she used a deductive approach to analyse her interview data.

> *Catherine:* The PhD came out of me wondering [why] everybody says that the non-profit sector is different. There are these assumptions embedded in all discourses and conversations about the sector that it is somehow different from the state or the market, and I accepted those assumptions for quite a long period of time until I started doing a PhD . . . so I was looking at an organisational space, a social space, that was large, complex, heterogeneous . . . a whole field of organisations known as the community sector or non-profit sector. So it's a lot of organisations, and I wanted to know why they were . . . different from organisations in the state and organisations in the market . . . this is

what people assumed. What I did first was have a look at a whole bunch of writing about the sector and about theorising around the sector and there's a lot of that emerging in the USA in particular—theories of the non-profit sector—and none of them answered the questions about why it was different. They all invoked this assumption of difference but never actually answered the questions, so I followed up a few references which took me to a body of organisational theory which . . . provides the theoretical justification for the perception of difference. So then I applied that theory to non-profit human service organisations in Queensland, and really it was to see whether or not this theoretical explanation for the assumption of difference held.

Robyn Munford and Jackie Sanders—Working successfully with families

Robyn Munford and Jackie Sanders used qualitative and quantitative strategies in a multi-phase study on what worked for families receiving family support services from a non-government child and family welfare agency in New Zealand. The research was conducted with the support of Barnardos New Zealand and the Foundation for Research, Science and Technology, New Zealand. The first stage involved an extensive file review of a twelve-month caseload for the whole organisation. The second stage primarily involved qualitative research—a small sample of families was intensively tracked as they moved through the service, and followed up three months after completion. Finally, a prospective statistical analysis of client and intervention factors over a twelve-month caseload was undertaken to analyse relationships between a wide range of factors and client change (Munford & Sanders, 1996, 1998, 1999). Jackie talks here about how the study originated.

Jackie: I was a Regional Director for Barnardos New Zealand and we were managing a large number of family support programs. I was keen to understand the ways in which our services might be contributing to family wel'.-being and also to understand more about the

13

possible long-term effects of our services on clients and their families. I also had an interest in understanding better the link between management styles and practice approaches in terms of identifying ways that the two can best be aligned for the greatest client gain. We had a link with Massey University which was probably more personal than anything—it being the place where I had done my Master's degree. We began dialogue with people in sociology and social work and Robyn was one of those people. We put together a working party to try to secure funding—this was successful and the rest, as they say, is history. We secured ongoing funding for four years to undertake a really detailed analysis of the family support program and as a result we were able to produce a very clear picture of the role of strengths-based work in family change and also to begin to understand more clearly the relationship between management styles and practice effectiveness. From that we developed an ongoing research partnership between Massey and Barnardos that has been successfully operating for six years now. I think we have an abiding interest in the complex mix of factors—personal client, structural, agency organisational, funding and practice—that combine together to generate good interventions for clients.

Dorothy Scott—Identification of post-partum depression

Dorothy talks here about the background to this study (1987a, 1987b, 1992).

> *Dorothy:* I was working as a social worker in a psychiatric ward of the Queen Victoria Hospital in Melbourne in the late 1970s and early 1980s and I was very involved in the treatment of women with post-partum psychiatric conditions. It gradually dawned on me that women with depressive disorders, unlike those with acute psychotic disorders, seemed to be admitted to hospital very late—long after serious depressive symptoms had

developed and often after real damage had been done to the mother–infant relationship and the couple relationship. So I became interested in how primary health care workers like maternal and child health nurses might be able to identify post-partum depression and make earlier referrals. I enrolled in a Master's degree and for my thesis I intended to develop a simple instrument for the nurses to identify post-partum depression and test it for its validity and reliability—a very traditional research project really, which others have subsequently done with the Edinburgh Post-Natal Depression Instrument. But it didn't turn out as I intended. The nurses told me that they didn't have a mandate to do mental-state examinations on mothers— that women came to see them to have their babies weighed and measured and that the mothers were highly sensitive to nurses prying into private issues such as their emotional state. In my literature search I also read an article on a study on anxiety among mothers of young babies and when I followed it up and spoke with the researcher she told me that the nurses had discarded that instrument as soon as the research was finished! There seemed little point in developing an instrument which nurses were not prepared to use. So instead I thought it might be useful to observe at length how nurses who were regarded by their peers as being particularly skilled in their interpersonal skills went about assessing women for depression. I suppose we would see it today as describing 'best practice'. I also wanted to understand the norms which governed the interaction between the nurse and the mother, and to interview mothers about what they saw as the role of the nurse and what they might find acceptable in regard to the nurse exploring issues related to their emotional well-being. So I used a number of methods—direct observation of three purposively selected maternal and child health nurses at work, followed by in-depth interviews with the nurses, and semi-structured interviews with a mixture of closed and open-ended questions with a sample of 45 mothers in their homes. While I was doing the thesis I had two children of my own and so I was a client of the maternal and child health service myself, although my nurses were not in the study of course. But I kept notes on my own experiences of the service and although I had not intended these notes to be a data source, this added an informal participant-observation dimension to the study which ultimately proved to be extremely valuable in understanding the subtle nuances and 'unconscious dynamics' of the nurse–mother relationship. This research stimulated my curiosity about practice wisdom or clinical judgement and that has continued to be a great interest.

Cheryl Tilse—The long goodbye

This is a study of the experiences of older people who place a spouse in an aged care facility and the conditions of the facility which shape the nature of the experiences of visitors (Tilse, 1996). It involved several methods of data collection, including in-depth interviews, observation, semi-structured interviews and document analysis. We talk with Cheryl later about her use of observation, the usefulness of combining qualitative data collection approaches, analysing data, writing up and dissemination of findings.

> Cheryl: I was working as a research assistant on a large project looking at the social, emotional and economic costs of dementia and part of that had been semi-structured interviews with 243 people who were caring for a relative with dementia. I was particularly interested in the interviews I did with spouses who had placed a partner in a nursing home. I felt that the semi-structured interviews really hadn't captured just how traumatic the experience was for them. So I became very interested in understanding what it was all about from their perspective . . . I was particularly concerned about what happens to people who've been married for 50, 60 years when they have this involuntary separation, when one partner goes into a nursing home. I was interested in following their experiences and understanding what it was like for them to try and continue

or exit from the marriage within an organisational setting. So I was also concerned about the context in which they visited, the purpose of meeting and visiting and how nursing homes provided for family visiting and so on . . . I was determined to try and catch what it was like for the older people . . . My concern was that their perspective wasn't understood in practice or in policy. Visitors were being constructed in policy as resources to help the organisation and to provide resources for the resident, and I had a very firm view that the purpose and meaning of visiting for this group was particularly different.

Comments

Several points about qualitative research emerge from these examples. First, it is important to note that each of these studies grew out of a particular time and place. For example, Tim and Wendy Booth's study can be seen in the context of the history of deinstitutionalisation and the emergence of reproductive rights for people with intellectual disabilities. Similarly, Anne Coleman's study is about a particular community of homeless people in a particular area that was undergoing urban redevelopment and gentrification at a particular period of time. Cheryl Tilse's study was a response to what she considered to be a too-narrow conception of the role of spouse visitors in nursing homes.

One of the issues for qualitative research is therefore the degree of generalisability of findings across settings. The researcher needs to acknowledge the limitation of their study's findings in terms of the context in which they were obtained and give the reader sufficient information about this context. The reader needs to be aware of this so that they can make allowances when extrapolating the findings to other settings.

Second, it is probably obvious to the reader that the sample size in most of these studies is much smaller than one would expect in quantitative research and that the sample is often not selected systematically to ensure that it is representative of a particular population. Obtaining representative samples in these contexts is often very difficult, and as the researcher seeks greater depth of understanding there is an inevitable trade-off in the number of people able to be included in the study. This also places limits on generalisability. However, if one considers the unit of attention as the phenomenon under investigation, rather than the number of individuals, then the sample is often much larger than first appears. Thus in the studies of Anne Coleman, Cheryl Tilse or Robyn Munford and Jackie Sanders, the number of interactions or contacts investigated would have been infinitely larger than the number of individuals or families involved.

Third, we can see from these examples that in qualitative inquiry the researcher cannot be and should not be written out of the text. This relates to the development of the research question and, as we shall see, it permeates all parts of the qualitative research process. The qualitative researcher is inextricably immersed in the research; thus qualitative research requires a high level of 'reflexivity' or self-reflection about one's part in the phenomenon under study. For some qualitative researchers the questions they explore grow out of a strong ideological commitment and the pursuit of social justice. Some qualitative researchers are happy to acknowledge this and discuss their role in terms of 'positioning', arguing that all claims to knowledge are situated and partial (Marcus, 1994). This may give the research its driving force and provide an entrée into particular social worlds—but there is also a risk that the researcher may avoid finding what they do not want or do not expect to find.

For the reader interested in generating their own research questions, we would suggest that the conception of the question is usually not too difficult for those curious about the world around them and it may be more difficult choosing which of many questions to explore. For some, it is a matter of recognising that they already have questions waiting to be crystallised and that the task is one of noticing the questions embedded in the conversations they have about their work with themselves or others.

Developing the embryonic question into a researchable form is more difficult and in qualitative research the question(s) may continue to be refined throughout the whole study. This is where it is important to have others, preferably not too closely involved with the site of the research, who can act as a sounding board on how the question is best framed, as this will shape how it can be investigated.

It is also important to discover what other research has already been done in relation to the question. Some important material may exist only in the form of unpublished reports, which have to be tracked down through a network of people, organisations and peak bodies or clearing houses.

It is highly desirable to undertake a thorough literature search and here the assistance of a specialist librarian will be helpful in accessing the numerous electronic databases which contain the published research literature. This involves carefully selecting key words relating to the research topic and systematically searching electronic data bases for books, journal articles and reports which have been classified according to one or more of the key words. It is possible to pay someone to do this for you, but it is essential that this person fully understand your question and your setting and thus it is preferable to do it together. That way you also learn the skills of searching the literature.

It is important to be aware that the same thing may be described differently in different places and sometimes the same terminology means rather different things in different places. For example, the term 'child care' in Australia generally refers to the day care of children of working parents, whereas in the United Kingdom 'child care' is often synonymous with child welfare or child protection. If the literature search is crossing service systems, or is going back to a time when different terminology prevailed, then it is obviously important to know the range of terms to use in any literature search.

More challenging again is to ask 'What is my question a question of?' in order to conceptualise your issue of interest. What you are interested in may be a concrete example of a broader phenomenon and it may be very useful to consult this broader literature. For example, in the study described above on post-natal depression and the role of the maternal and child health nurse, asking 'What is the question a question of?' led to a body of literature which a literature search based on the more obvious key words would not have accessed.

By conceptualising the question as one which was essentially about the core and marginal functions of a professional role (the core role of the nurse was weighing and measuring babies and the marginal role was assessing maternal emotional well-being), role theory became a central conceptual framework for the study. It led to examining other studies which at first sight might seem totally irrelevant (such as studies on the roles of policewomen and parish priests). These, however, proved to be very pertinent and helped lead the researcher out of a narrow mindset to fresh ways of seeing the issue.

Research is essentially all about seeing the world in fresh ways, about searching again or re-searching the same territory and seeing it in a different light. In qualitative research we are particularly interested in how others see and experience the world. This requires us to be very aware of the lens which we bring to the task. Perhaps it is a perceptual impossibility to look at one's own lens at the same time as one is looking through it, but this is one of the many fascinating challenges of qualitative research. The excitement resides not so much in reaching the destination, for we can never completely enter the world of the other, but in the voyage and what might be found on the way. The swampy lowlands await you.

2

Ethics and organisations

The best one can do is to consider the ethical and political issues in asking a particular research question, determine the areas of concern prior to the research, take into account professional standards that have been established and then consider the ethics of the entire research process as an individual case with its own social and political ramifications (Minichiello et al., 1990, pp. 245–6).

It may seem strange to combine ethics and organisational issues, yet in qualitative research in the human services, perhaps more than in any other area of research, doing the right thing by research participants coexists with the pragmatic process of 'getting in, getting on and getting out' of the research setting.

The ethical principles which should guide research are fairly clear. Both professional ethics and research ethics are based on similar core principles, such as beneficence and duty of care, and so one might assume that there will be clear and congruent criteria for determining ethical behaviour in research in the human services. Yet standard research and practice ethics statements let us down simply because they are designed from different perspectives with different ends in sight: the academic development of knowledge on one hand, the delivery of service on the other. They are not designed for the interface of these two domains.

In this chapter it is argued that there are complex issues which arise in research in the human services, particularly when the boundaries between practitioner and researcher roles, and those between the roles of client and research subject, become blurred. The interconnectedness between the ethics and the politics of research is evident at every stage of the research process with the most fundamental question being 'Who owns the research?'. From how some questions come to be framed as questions for inquiry to the ways in which research findings are disseminated and utilised, the process is shaped by the interests and relative power of the various stakeholders. For example, the interests and power of agency management, service providers and clients may differ. These players also exist within a social and political context. The prevailing orthodoxy can allow certain questions to be asked and not others. The political significance of a social problem will influence the priority given to it in research funding, the manner in which its findings are received and how its recommendations are implemented.

Gaining ethics approval for qualitative research

In the past decade or so there has been an increasing awareness of the complex ethical issues associated with research involving humans and animals. Examples of grossly unethical practices involving human experimentation in medical research led to the development of mechanisms aimed at protecting the interests of participants. Research grants and the permission to undertake research under the auspices of one or another organisation are increasingly subject to processes under which the ethical issues associated with a particular study are screened by institutional ethics committees, sometimes known as ethics review boards. While the core principles governing the decision-making of these bodies are similar, they vary considerably in their operations, requirements and procedures. Prospective researchers should familiarise themselves with the specific requirements of the relevant ethics body very early on when considering a research project.

Human research ethics committees play an important gate-keeping role in all research involving human subjects and are likely to be extra vigilant in their consideration of proposals for research concerning any potentially vulnerable groups of people. Ethics committees have a duty to consider all possible sources of harm and satisfy themselves that the researcher has thought through all the relevant issues prior to granting permission to proceed. The onus is firmly on the researcher to show that the proposed research will not cause harm and that adequate safeguards are put in place to ensure this. Even when practitioner researchers are experienced in working with a particular group which may be considered vulnerable in the research context, they will still have to demonstrate to an ethics committee that they have the appropriate skills to undertake the proposed research with this group.

While ethical guidelines used in university and medical research settings were originally oriented to biomedical experimentation, as in clinical drug trials, their mandate has now extended to behavioural and social science research. Ethics review boards are often unfamiliar with qualitative research and this can create difficulties for researchers, particularly in the field of health. Attempts are now being made to assist medical and health research ethics review boards to develop a better understanding of qualitative research and its associated ethical issues. For example, in Australia the National Health and Medical Research Council has produced a special paper on ethical aspects of qualitative methods in health research (National Health and Medical Research Council, 1995).

Some of the most common areas of misunderstanding in relation to qualitative research relate to the often small sample size and the lack of specific hypotheses, control groups and predetermined questions, which can lead to the false assumption that the proposed study is not sufficiently rigorous. It is therefore important to address such concerns directly in any proposal.

Institutional ethics committees may also be unfamiliar with the human service field, so those undertaking qualitative research in the human services can encounter a double-layered lack of understanding. Ethics review boards may not appreciate that the study is part and parcel of professional practice, governed by professional ethics and under the auspices of an organisation with its own structure of accountability. Thus, for example, workers who routinely collect feedback from service users may find that the ethics review board is uneasy about such data being collected from people who are dependent upon the service and as a consequence may be seen as constrained in their capacity to give freely their informed consent.

The boundary between a clinical audit or quality assurance project in an agency and 'research' may also appear blurred. In our experience this is less likely to be a problem with medical ethics review boards than with university-based ethics committees in the behavioural and social sciences, as the distinction is usually better understood in health settings. In university-auspiced research in the human services it is usually necessary to have the permission of both the university ethics committee and the relevant human services organisation(s), with the latter typically being one of the prerequisites for the former.

Outside universities and hospitals the accountability mechanisms for research are still developing and research in some areas remains relatively unregulated. In some human services agencies, there may not be an agency policy or set of guidelines on research and those wishing to undertake research may unwittingly find themselves in an ethical minefield. Other organisations, such as government departments, may be concerned with the potential political ramifications of the research and at times research proposals may be thwarted, ostensibly on ethical grounds.

Some human service agencies are accelerating their efforts to provide guidelines and structures to manage ethical research. An excellent model of how this can be done is that of the Australian child and family welfare agency Uniting Care Burnside. This agency has produced a Research Code of Ethics (Burnside, 2000) which can be copied in its entirety for non-profit purposes. It covers all types of research, including quantitative and qualitative studies, and is particularly focused on safeguards for research with vulnerable children and young people. It takes the prospective researcher through the research process and sets out clear guidelines in relation to designing valid research, obtaining voluntary informed consent, implementing the research, protecting privacy, maximising benefits and disseminating the research results.

Qualitative research in the human services poses particular challenges in relation to ethical considerations. This chapter focuses on three main issues: informed consent; intrusiveness; and confidentiality.

> The characteristics of qualitative investigation seem to generate particular decision-making problems for the investigator who seeks to safeguard the research participant. There are three types of problems, although the categories are loose and overlapping: (a) the participant–investigator relationship itself, within which are divulged many confidences, (b) the investigator's subjective interpretation of the collected data, and (c) the more loosely defined, emergent, design (Ramos, 1989, p. 58).

Informed consent

The capacity of an individual to give freely their informed consent to research is a core principle in research ethics; it is a capacity that can be diminished by a range of factors. One factor that is commonly mentioned in research ethical guidelines is that of incentives. It is common to reimburse research participants for any out-of-pocket expenses in the human services but the notion of voluntary consent is sometimes thought to be diminished if undue enticement exists in the form of payment. On the other hand, some organisations which routinely undertake social research with low-income families, such as the Brotherhood of St Laurence in Melbourne, have a policy of reimbursing research participants on the ground that their time and knowledge is valued. The researcher therefore needs to think through the issue in the context of their specific project and consider what might constitute undue enticement for particular participants.

A central issue in human service research is the complications which arise when the researcher is also the service provider, as the capacity of a client to withhold consent can be diminished by the unequal power and the dependency typically entailed in the worker–client relationship. Even where the researcher is not the client's worker, similar complexities might arise when the research is being undertaken on behalf of, or in association with, the agency from which the client is receiving a service, as the person may be apprehensive about the possible withdrawal of the service if they refuse to participate.

In some instances the agency commissions research and the relationship between the agency and the researcher is governed by a contract. Even if the research is externally funded, the researcher may be located in an organisation such as a university which has close links and an interdependent relationship with the agency. For example, university departments that provide professional education may be dependent upon the agency for the provision of much-needed field placements for their students. Such factors can and do influence the research process, and it is important that arrangements of this kind do not adversely affect the interests of research participants.

Thus, the researcher has a clear obligation to inform potential research subjects that their access to services will not be affected whether they agree to participate in the research or not, and that they are free to withdraw from the research at any time. Most ethics guidelines require that this be stated in writing and that the research participant signs to the effect that they understand these conditions. For people whose comprehension of English is limited, this agreement should be provided in their own language. Some people, by virtue of their age, cognitive capacity or the fact that they are statutory clients or involuntary patients, have a diminished capacity to give informed consent. These are often the very people with whom human services are involved and whose input to the service providers and managers is sought through qualitative research.

Under conditions in which it is likely that the capacity for freely given informed consent may be diminished, researchers have an additional duty of care to potential participants. For example, subjects should not be asked to give consent to things which could harm them. It has been argued that: 'Regardless of the information divulged, research participants should be able to trust the investigator to protect their welfare. The depth of this trust should increase in proportion to the degree of shared intimacy and respondent vulnerability' (Ramos, 1989, p. 59).

Research subjects, like clients, have a right to be informed of any limitations on the confidentiality of what they may divulge to the researcher. This can raise particularly complex issues for researchers who, as a result of legal requirements, agency policy or professional ethics, might be obliged in certain circumstances to divulge information. For example, the researcher may have a duty of care to third parties such as children in child protection research.

In relation to children, there are additional issues and it is perhaps not surprising that the voices of children have remained largely inaudible as a result. A central issue in any research involving children is to what extent, if any, they are capable of giving informed consent and under what circumstances and to what degree parents can give consent on their behalf. Prospective researchers should be aware of any legislation which relates to minors in their particular context.

> Generally speaking, minors under the age of eighteen cannot enter into binding contracts . . . Where children are to be involved in such research and are too young for their consent to be legally meaningful, either or both parents can exercise their powers as guardians to do so (Commonwealth Department of Human Services and Health, 1995, p. 90).

Yet a minor's capacity for informed consent is dependent upon age and individual maturity, and older children and adolescents may well be in a position to express their opinion about participating in research. Parental permission does not justify overriding a child's or young person's opposition to participation, so it may be appropriate for researchers to seek the views of both parents and children. There are limits to which parents can give consent in relation to their children's participation in research, and this is related to the potential harm or benefit which the research might involve for the child.

In medical research, a distinction has been made between 'therapeutic' and 'non-therapeutic research' in relation to children as subjects. Therapeutic research is intended to benefit the research subject directly and has traditionally been regarded as having lower requirements in regard to obtaining consent, and allowing higher levels of risk, than non-therapeutic research, in which there is no direct potential benefit. In regard to research in which the proposed benefit might accrue to those other than the subjects, the question remains: 'Is it ethical to use children in research which is for the "social good", even if parents give their permission?' (Koocher & Keith-Speigel 1994, p. 51).

The US Department of Health and Human Services has stated that research may be acceptable on children under such conditions as long as the research poses 'no greater than minimal risk'.

> Minimal Risk means that the risks of harm anticipated in the proposed research are not greater, considering probability and magnitude, than those ordinarily encountered in daily life or during the performance of routine physical or psychological examinations or tests (HHS, 1983, quoted in Koocher & Keith-Speigel, 1994, p. 51).

Such a definition is ambiguous and is ultimately a matter of judgement by researchers and ethics bodies. The need to assess the possible risks involved in participating in research applies to adults as well as children, as there is a clear duty to inform potential subjects in research of the possible adverse effects of participation. Yet it is not easy to assess the level of risk, as much depends on the characteristics of the client and the psychological significance of the data being sought.

Communicating the purpose of research to children also requires skilful adaptation of the processes used for adults. In a recent UK study of children who had been adopted when they were five years

27

or older (Thomas et al., 1999), children whose adoptive parents had given their permission were provided with both a leaflet and an audio cassette explaining the study. The leaflet had photographs of the researchers and used simple language, short sentences, a large typeface and colour graphics. The audio cassette enabled the children to hear the researchers' voices and to form some impression of the people who might interview them, and proved to be particularly useful for children who had limited literacy or who did not enjoy reading. We interviewed Caroline Thomas, and parts of that interview are included in the chapters on tailoring research to specific groups (Chapter 5), data analysis (Chapter 7) and the shift from research back to practice (Chapter 9).

Intrusiveness

Qualitative research methods such as in-depth interviewing and observation can be highly intrusive. People are often interviewed about highly personal matters, sometimes relating to loss and trauma. In some human service fields this applies to almost the entire client population.

> Research on child abuse and neglect generally involves domains that are consensually regarded as private. Such work is commonly perceived as more intrusive than researchers believe it to be . . . Research on child maltreatment may be susceptible to the research analogue to iatrogenic effects in treatment. For example, if, as some clinicians believe, repeated interviewing about an experience of victimisation induces further trauma, there is an obvious conflict with the need to gather information for research . . . are the anxiety, increased scrutiny, and perhaps even self-fulfilling prophecy that may result warranted by the knowledge to be gained? (Melton & Flood, 1994, pp. 23–24).

Such risks can be reduced, but not eliminated, by using professionally trained interviewers who are sensitive to the needs of subjects in the way they conduct interviews. However, it may also be necessary to make available to interviewees opportunities to debrief after the research interview, and access to appropriate services should be arranged in the planning stage of the study. Many ethics review boards now regard this as a precondition for approving some projects.

Observational methods can also be very intrusive. The presence of an observer or the awareness that the interview is being observed through a one-way screen or recorded on film can affect the phenomenon under investigation. This is not just a methodological concern—it is also a serious ethical issue. As a result of the observation a service provider may have a heightened performance anxiety which may affect the quality of service offered, or the client's anxiety might affect their ability to make use of what is being provided.

While the intrusiveness of such qualitative research methods is very obvious, even 'unobtrusive' research about which the individual may remain unaware, for instance, the perusal of case files or official records, can constitute a serious violation of privacy. Thus, whenever records are used for purposes other than that for which they were originally intended, it is important to think through the ethical questions involved. Who should have access to this material? Is client permission necessary or will agency permission suffice? Would document-based research be feasible if the permission of all relevant parties had to be obtained?

Confidentiality

At first sight confidentiality seems a fairly straightforward ethical issue, and in the research literature is almost exclusively dealt with in terms of developing data collection and storage systems in which it is not possible to identify the research subjects. Accordingly, research participants are routinely given assurances of confidentiality. But in qualitative research this is not always so simple.

In research that is based on a case study method, whether the case be a community, an organisation or a family, it can sometimes be difficult to disguise the data so that the setting or participants are completely unrecognisable, particularly to those familiar with the field. To reduce the risk of recognition, it is possible to present data in a disaggregated way, such as presenting interviewees' responses to different questions or issues under theme-based headings. One of the dilemmas of reporting qualitative research is, however, that if the purpose of the research is to show the phenomenon in a holistic way, disaggregating the data can weaken its essence.

Should other researchers have access to the data in order to undertake secondary analysis? Being prepared to allow one's research data to be analysed by others is regarded as an important safeguard against fraudulent research, and secondary data analysis is very useful as it can allow subsequent investigation of valuable data in relation to different research questions. For these reasons researchers are usually required to keep their data for a number of years to enable others to have access to it. In contract research the data typically belongs to those funding the research and thus future access is not controlled by those actually doing the research. This can create problems when applied to qualitative research as 'later use by different researchers may be inappropriate for projects which collected in-depth interviews on sensitive topics' (Commonwealth Department of Human Services and Health, 1995, p. 14).

Even when the researcher 'owns' the data, once the research is part of the public domain the researcher may have little control over how it is used and aspects may be selectively quoted. 'Researchers noted that it was frequently difficult to control the use of reports once they became a part of the public domain. They expressed concerns about simplistic or sensationalist media coverage' (Commonwealth Department of Human Services and Health, 1995, p. 13).

Researchers must therefore be aware that what they write may be used in ways other than they intended. For a research participant to see their words used or, as they might perceive it, misused, in the public domain can be a deeply violating experience even if their identity is not revealed.

To disguise the verbatim quotes of interviewees by paraphrasing them would defeat the purpose of much qualitative research. The challenge then is to disseminate the voices of those previously unheard in the public domain in ways in which privacy is protected. The researchers doing the older adopted children study described above did this in a novel way (Thomas et al., 1999). They tape-recorded other children reading the transcripts of the adopted children's interviews and played the interviews to prospective adoptive parents and social workers during their training sessions to enable them to appreciate the subjective experiences of adopted children in their own words. This protected the privacy of the adopted children while evocatively conveying their experiences much more powerfully than the written word allowed. This example highlights the sensitive and individualised ways in which researchers can apply ethical principles.

Ethical and political complexities of research within organisations

In the past the ethical issues associated with conducting qualitative research within human services organisations tended to be overlooked, yet issues in relation to informed consent, intrusiveness and confidentiality are equally as applicable to organisations and their staff as to their clients. Research has the capacity to harm the legitimate interests of the organisation and the professional and personal reputations of the individuals it employs. Research can also consume valuable organisational resources such as staff time. Traditionally in the social sciences this has been seen as a political issue—the problem of 'getting in, getting on and getting out'. In one study, researchers intent on exposing the practices of staff in psychiatric institutions posed as patients to gain entry, with little consideration given to their obligations to the staff or to the organisation (Rosenhan, 1973).

There is a growing awareness these days of the ethical implications of such research. Doing research in institutions today entails much more careful negotiation of the respective rights and responsibilities of the organisation and the researcher. Human services organisations are increasingly sensitive to the political ramifications of research, perhaps to a degree that will make such research more difficult to undertake in the future. Just as researchers once regarded what are now seen as legitimate ethical issues as merely political issues, there is a risk that some organisations may reframe political issues as ethical issues in order to minimise adverse public exposure as a result of legitimate inquiry.

Few qualitative researchers have described in detail the ethical and political processes of 'getting in, getting on and getting out' of their research settings. Kelley Johnson, who conducted an ethnographic study on intellectually disabled women living in an institution in Victoria in the early 1990s, is an exception. In this case, gaining the approval of staff initially proved more difficult than gaining the approval of senior management:

> . . . formal permission did not really 'get me in'. Staff at the institution had been under frequent attack from the media because of conditions in the institution and were defensive and resistant to the idea of my research. My decision during this time to base myself in the locked unit assisted in the process of 'getting in' . . . I was less of a threat to

other staff since most of my time was spent confined in one unit. I was effectively locked away (Johnson & Scott, 1997, p. 29).

'Getting in' is therefore not just a matter of gaining official approval but also of engaging staff at various levels of the organisation. This is perhaps particularly challenging when the research is initiated by the organisation itself or by a funding body for the purpose of evaluation. If it is a pilot program which is being evaluated, staff will often feel a heightened performance anxiety, particularly if the program is experiencing the normal teething problems. It is desirable to delay evaluation until after the initial implementation problems have been solved, but sometimes the funding source requires an evaluation to be built in from the outset. If this is so then an evaluation, be it a process or an outcome evaluation, needs to be placed in the context of its occurrence within the implementation phase of a new program. Even in an established program the staff may be apprehensive and hard to engage, due to their fear that management or the funding body has an ulterior motive and that the future of the program is under threat. Sometimes such fears are well founded.

Given that the interests of management and service providers might be quite different, the ethical question arises as to under what circumstances can the former give consent on behalf of the latter? There is very little in the literature on research ethics to guide the researcher in this territory. We would advise researchers to be honest in their communication with all parties and to develop transparent processes about informed consent, confidentiality and the possible impact of the research on participants.

It is not sufficient just to 'get in'. The researcher must also be able to 'get on' with research participants. From the perspective of staff, researchers can get in the way of people going about their normal work and are a potential source of interference. Issues relating to the degree of access which researchers have in the setting need to be clearly worked out and communicated to all of those concerned. Even where this has been carefully negotiated, events can unfold which threaten the research. While Kelley Johnson was undertaking her research a government decision was made to close the institution.

Once the decision was made to close the institution, my situation became for a short time, more difficult. Staff were angry at the closure and instituted industrial action bans which included the exclusion of all researchers from the site. The reciprocal nature of my involvement with the staff in the locked unit and the length of time I had been part of the institution led to a decision to revoke the ban for my research (Johnson & Scott, 1997, p. 30).

Interestingly, in the light of this change, Johnson became focused on the process of deinstitutionalisation, making her research a unique study of the impact of this policy shift on the intellectually disabled women, their families and the staff inside the institution. This brought added challenges, not the least being that the families thus became research participants as well. The researcher also became privy to the conflictual processes within the organisation as staff faced the loss of jobs and the uncertainty of the process of closure.

> . . . many of these families had put their own ambivalence and pain behind the walls of the locked unit with their relative. Now with the decision to close the institution, these feelings were released, and the existing processes of deinstitutionalisation did nothing to resolve them . . . the complexity of my study increased. I became involved in management meetings and in work with the people closing the institution. I found the gap between these encounters and life in the unit enormous. Because of the industrial disputes arising from the closure decision, I found myself privy to information from groups in conflict with each other (Johnson & Scott, 1997, p. 31).

It is fortunate that most qualitative studies in human service settings are not as challenging as Kelley Johnson's turned out to be, but all research conducted in organisations will present some difficulties as organisations are complex and dynamic sociopolitical worlds. Conducting research within such settings inevitably adds to their complexity.

> 'Getting out' also creates its ethical and political challenges. Issues about differences in interpretation also arise when feedback occurs before the report is completed. While the point of view of participants about a social process is important, it is also self-interested and embedded in the power relations of the community. The final interpretation has to rest with the researcher, except in action research in which discussion and negotiation are a part of the research design (Commonwealth Department of Human Services and Health 1995, p. 12).

Organisational researcher Richard Scott has identified the later stages of a study as being particularly likely to be fraught by such problems.

... misunderstandings between the researcher and his subjects often come to the surface on the occasion when the research findings are published . . . even the researcher who does not centre his analysis on deviations (from rules or ideals) of one sort or another may still offend his subjects simply by applying his particular perspective, for he attempts to take an objective and relative view of matters which from the standpoint of his subjects are value-laden and unique. How much and what sorts of things to tell subjects about the research in progress and how much and what sorts of things to put into the published report—these are the kinds of ethical questions to which the open field researcher will find no easy solutions (Scott, 1969, pp. 571–2).

While such issues are relevant in all social research, they are of critical importance in qualitative research in the human services. Feedback loops from the research to policy and practice will often be central to the research, and the tensions which may arise need to be anticipated and managed in an honest and open manner.

Stories from the field

While it is tempting to ask for clearer guidelines to assist researchers in their decision-making about ethical issues, it is illusory to think that there will be simple prescriptive solutions to the complex ethical and organisational dilemmas inherent in qualitative research in human services settings. Ultimately many of the dilemmas require individual judgements based on the characteristics of specific situations. Unfortunately there is a lack of case studies or detailed descriptive accounts of how different researchers have grappled with ethical issues in the research process.

The lack of such accounts may be partly due to the apprehension researchers feel about exposing their decisions 'warts and all' and leaving themselves open to criticism. We hope that the following first-hand accounts of how qualitative researchers have struggled with some of these issues may help others in their endeavours to conduct ethical qualitative research. After all, 'Ethics is not just a nice thing to have; research is fundamentally weak without it' (Deetz, 1985, p. 254).

In the following examples, the complexity and, at times, the interrelationship of ethical issues and organisational issues which can be involved in qualitative research in the human services are highlighted.

Dorothy Scott—Child protection assessment

Dorothy: In looking back on my PhD thesis on child protection assessment what strikes me are the unanticipated ethical and political issues which arose as well as the fact that the issues I had anticipated proved to be more complex and more difficult to handle than I had expected. This was partly because of my close connections with the hospital setting in which the research was conducted yet without those close connections it is unlikely that I would have been able to do the research at all. At the time I undertook the research I was not working there but I had previously acted as a clinical consultant and group supervisor to the unit in which the research was based, and so I had close relationships with many of the staff.

I used in-depth interviews and observation to intensively shadow a small number of alleged child abuse cases through the hospital unit, a statutory child protection agency and the police. I repeatedly interviewed professionals involved with the same families throughout the life of the case, focusing on the factors to which they were attending in their assessment. Where possible I also observed episodes of practice, ranging from observing interviews with children through a one-way screen in the hospital unit, accompanying child protection workers on home visits to attending staff meetings, case conferences and court hearings. I interviewed the parents in their home three months after the cessation of contact with the services.

Obtaining the informed consent of parents proved to be a more complex ethical issue than I had anticipated. At the point at which each case was selected, the parents in this study were in the immediate aftermath of discovering that their child might have been physically or sexually abused. While no parent was a statutory client at the time they gave their consent to the study, several parents became the subject of a child protection investigation and others later expressed their fear of becoming so. Some parents were clearly in a state of crisis. In light of this, I chose to delay approaching these parents in the immediate crisis in order to avoid seeking parental consent at a time when their capacity for informed judgement might be most compromised. This entailed forgoing the collection of data in the initial phase of the case, thus illustrating the 'trade-off' which can occur between ethical and methodological priorities.

There were other 'trade-offs' of this nature. For example, I decided not to tape-record interviews or to interview parents before their involvement with the various services had finished, both significant methodological sacrifices, because of the risk that parents might divulge information which could be subpoenaed in legal proceedings. The decision not to give parents the option of being interviewed throughout the period of service involvement was seen by some of my colleagues as paternalistic and disempowering. My reason was that it might be very hard for parents to trust the confidentiality of what they might say to me when they knew that I was in close contact and on first-name terms with the professionals they were seeing. This may be an example of 'justified paternalism'.

All of the children in my study were aged ten years or less, and parental permission was sought to observe hospital social workers' interviews with the children through a one-way screen. This was a standard practice in the hospital service and colleagues, trainees and clinical supervisors routinely observed interviews in this way (with the permission of the parent and the knowledge of the child). I did not seek parental permission to interview the children as I felt that interviewing the children could not be justified due to the risk of further traumatisation. While the potential risks could not be quantified, nor could the potential benefits.

However, as the study unfolded, the issue of children's involvement in the research became less clear cut. For example, on several occasions in the follow-up home interviews with parents the children were unexpectedly present for some of the interview although I had arranged with the parents to visit at a time when the children would not be there. As it happened, the situations were resolved by parents deciding to put the children to bed or arranging other activities, but this does illustrate some of the unanticipated complexities of naturalistic studies involving children.

While I had rejected the possibility of interviewing children because of the potential harm this might cause, I saw observation through a one-way screen as having a much lower level of intrusiveness and risk. In part this belief was shaped by it being routine practice in the hospital for colleagues to view interviews through a one-way screen. It was hard to assess the level of intrusiveness and risk for a particular child entailed in observation. For example, for some children it may have a marked impact on their capacity to express their feelings and make use of the therapeutic opportunity. Just because others were observing the interviews for non-research purposes does not, however, necessarily justify it.

In seeking consent from the parents for the observation of interviews with their child, I informed them that I planned to be present during all the interviews and that if, for some unexpected reason, I was unable to attend, their social worker would tell them of my absence. In relation to the child, however, I accepted the way each social worker generally managed the issue of observation. Some social workers routinely informed the child at the initial interview that sometimes there would be people behind the window and did not mention it again, while others informed the child on each occasion and even showed them the observation room and introduced them to those observing. Although I was uncomfortable watching interviews in which I was unsure whether the child was aware of being observed, it is possible that the more comfortable I felt, the more intrusive the observation may have been and the greater its effect on the interview.

In relation to the informed consent of colleagues, a difference between [my] understanding of what the social workers had agreed to and their understanding of what they had agreed to emerged late in the study. For example, in relation to the hospital social workers [I] believed that they understood that I would be observing intake meetings to describe how a case and other agencies involved were perceived. Yet when I presented my preliminary findings to the team some social workers expressed concern that I had drawn on all that I had observed and heard during intake meetings while they had believed that I was only at the intake meeting to 'pick up a new case'. I had very openly taken detailed notes throughout all of the intake meetings [that] included negative 'off the cuff' comments social workers and others had made about clients and other agencies. This type of data was very significant to the research questions. This placed me in a dilemma. Should data be used which some subjects believed was obtained under false pretences, even if this was not done so deliberately? Alternatively, was the objection an attempt to restrict academic freedom, and would not using the data compromise the integrity of the research? The matter was resolved, probably not to the satisfaction of either party, by removing the verbatim quotations and substituting paraphrasing of their comments.

Another ethical issue which unexpectedly arose was 'researcher as whistle-blower'—whether it was appropriate for me to intervene in a situation in which malpractice appeared to have occurred. In one case a 10-year-old boy was coercively removed from his family by child protection authorities in a way which appeared both unethical and illegal. While he had already been returned home by the stage I became involved, as the hospital social worker had intervened to secure this, if she had not done so should I have taken on this role? If I had, would I have endangered the study? If I hadn't, would I have been colluding with injustice?

Confidentiality also proved to be a more complex issue than I had originally anticipated. As the research progressed, I become increasingly aware of the difficulty of presenting the findings of research based on an intensive analysis of cases without using illustrations which [might] be recognisable to the staff and/or the clients themselves. The study specifically explored parents' perceptions of the services, and inter-organisational interactions, which meant that much of the data related to the often negative perceptions research subjects had in relation to one another. Can it be said that confidentiality has been preserved when a service provider might recognise a case in which she or he was involved and be able to identify the clients or other service providers whose perceptions about them and their agency are presented? What might be the consequences of this, real or imagined, for future interactions between the participants? My research [thus] generated many questions of an ethical and political nature, some of which cut across both of these categories, but few answers!

Anne Coleman—Five star motels

We introduced Anne Coleman's (2001) study of homelessness in Fortitude Valley in Chapter 1. In her interview with us, Anne reflected on the process of negotiating her entry into that particular community of homeless people. While this is very different from negotiating with a formal organisation, as in the example above, the issue of being an insider and/or outsider was still central. While she was an outsider in the sense that she was not a homeless person, she had lived and worked in the Valley and so was known to many homeless people in that community.

Anne: I lived in the area for about three years and this had overlapped with when I first started to work there . . . I knew that in a sense the insider bit was my entree into that community and I knew that it would probably overcome [problems] . . . there are a lot of documented things in methodologies about work with homeless people, about how tricky they are with outsiders. A fellow who had tried to do some work in the inner city about fifteen years before had actually not been able to do it and he said that he felt the

39

people were deliberately playing with him. Like they'd tell him one thing on Monday and on Wednesday they would tell him something else that was totally contradictory and he just couldn't negotiate that at all.

I also knew that . . . there were a couple of worries for me in the insider position . . . I was accepted to some extent in that community but I was never a complete insider. For example . . . at one stage someone said, 'Why don't you go and sleep out?' And I thought about it but it seemed almost hypocritical to me because even if I slept out for one night or if I slept out for two months, the reality was that as soon as it got too horrible or I'd had enough I still had a home to go to and I'd just say, 'See you all later fellas', and off I'd go. That not only seemed hypocritical, but also something that they would really call me on.

I guess in the end the only way I could conceptualise it was I had to move a bit past the insider/outsider [dichotomy] and I had to come to . . . a continuum conceptualisation where sometimes I was both of those things and I moved along the line constantly. And although that seems a bit at odds with a lot of what's written in methodology about insiders/outsiders, my feeling about it was really shored up by work I had done with people . . . I suppose an example of that stuff is that if you work with indigenous people the relationship [between you] can become quite strong and I think an element of that is that you're seen as being a valued person in the community. If you value them [in return] it's a very powerful thing when you work with them. When you do that, the relationship becomes unbelievably close . . . and probably in terms of white social work it would look like a very borderline unprofessional kind of relationship because of that closeness and involvement. At the same time, if you hurt somebody unintentionally, if you stepped on very sensitive ground, if you made a promise that you didn't keep, if you did what people perceived as 'playing games with them', you would immediately be moved—not move yourself—by people along that line from insider to outsider. So, within a split second you could go from being 'sister' to being 'that white bitch'—it would be that quick and it would be that total and both of those positions would be 100 per cent heartfelt and sincerely held.

So, I guess because I'd worked in that environment for a long time, that idea that I would move along the continuum all the way through this research sat quite well and in fact I think that's probably what allowed me to deal with some tricky stuff sometimes . . . something would happen . . . often not necessarily directly connected with me. It could be somebody had heard that they'd been talked about at a meeting in a derogatory way or I got quite a bit of stick when the Council closed off a set of stairs where Murri homeless people had sat and put up a barricade and then eventually put up a mural, an indigenous mural that was painted by other people. I copped quite a lot of stick around that time . . . people were very angry and there was no one else official to voice that to . . . they knew that I was interested in all of this stuff because that was the topic of my thesis . . . I was seen for both those reasons as being the appropriate person in that case. So, in that case I think it was my insider/outsider status that it was about.

And I think that a lot of what people told me was for that reason too. 'You're close enough for us to trust and we know that you won't let us down badly. We've watched you over ten years, but we also know you talk to those other people and we want you to tell them about this' . . . I think all the way through they were pretty clear that the research per se was for me but I think they probably trusted me that they would get something out of it in the end.

Angelina Yuen-Tsang —Social support networks of Chinese working mothers in Beijing

Angelina is a Hong Kong-based researcher who is investigating social support in mainland China—what constitutes help, and under what circumstances will people receive help from outside and from their peers and their family members. Her research was published in 1997 as *Towards a Chinese Conception of Social Support: A Study on the Social Support Networks of Chinese Working Mothers in Beijing*. This is a study of individuals and families within a particular community and issues relating to gaining the trust of the community were also central for Angelina. We talk with Angelina again later about her data collection and analysis processes. Here, she talks about how she needed to engage with those holding formal authority as well as make informal connections with people at the local level.

> *Angelina:* I believe in living in the community while doing participant observation, and I feel that if I am not immersed in that particular community's life, I cannot understand their way of thinking. So I had to find a place where I could stay, where I could live and have access to the people that I would like to interview . . . it took about a year to negotiate entry into one particular community . . . I didn't want to rush things because I felt that if I was to do a successful piece of grounded theory research, I had to fit into that community and that community had to receive me . . . And so I looked around in Beijing to try to find the community that was the best fit . . . I visited several communities and talked with the local officials, but I didn't just talk to the high officials. I talked to the middle level and then the front-line level to see whether I could click with them.
>
> I finally decided on the Fuguo community because I found that the local officials received me very well and didn't treat me as an external researcher intruding into their community. They received me very naturally. I found that they were treating me as just an ordinary academic who would like to know more about their community and there was no big deal about my particular research . . . I don't want to be followed all the time and I don't want to be treated as a VIP. I don't want to be given all the cases which are very special . . . cases from the very good families . . .

Yvonne: To what extent were you treated as an insider or an outsider? Were you always an outsider or did you develop more of an insider status over time?

Angelina: I think to the local officials I always remained as an outsider . . . but to the people in the community—because I'm hanging around the community, living in the community, shopping in the community—some of them treated me as a teacher from Hong Kong. So, sort of an insider/outsider because they knew that I was from Hong Kong but they treated me as a friend—a friendly researcher.

Robyn Munford and Jackie Sanders—Working successfully with families

We introduced Robyn and Jackie's research on family support services in New Zealand in Chapter 1. This was a large project, involving academic and community partnerships and a diverse research team of academics, practitioners and community members. In addition to the research reports (Munford et al., 1996, 1998; Sanders et al., 1999), other publications arising from this research include two papers on ethical issues in qualitative research with families (Munford & Sanders, 2000a; Munford & Sanders, 2000b) and a textbook on family support work (Munford & Sanders, 1999). We asked Robyn and Jackie to talk about the composition and functioning of the research team as well as well as some of the ethical and organisational issues they encountered.

Dorothy: Could you say something about your research team—the different roles which people had, the cultural mix, how it evolved and the changes that occurred in the team over time? What it was like for each of you to be part of this research team?

Robyn: Well, I am very clear that this research would not happen without the full-time efforts of a researcher [Jackie's role]. Jackie keeps the team on track and pushes the deadlines—all teams need this. Jackie and I are the longest-serving members of the team and have maintained the consistency as others have come and gone. I believe the secret of the success of the research is the team and the commitment to team meetings and clarity around tasks. Goals are set and reviewed and members are clear about their roles. We are now fortunate to have on our team community members who are part of the agencies we are researching. We also have a mix of cultures and experience and this adds to the diversity. We continually review our individual contributions to the team and reflect on progress to date.

Jackie: We have been really lucky to have ongoing funding and I think Robyn is right—without someone whose job it is to keep the research going, research like this will often fall by the wayside. There are a lot of challenges, particularly in managing the relationships with service delivery staff and with funders, that really require someone's constant attention. If this is added on to an already demanding job, say in teaching or practice, then it is always going to fall off the bottom of the list. We have really worked on the concept of teamwork and I feel are now at a point where we have a clear understanding of what being a team means. We have three people who are committed to completing the research. By this I mean the research as an activity is a central part of their working week. Two of us are employed part time with research money, and the other one, Robyn, is just amazingly dedicated to this process and has had an ongoing commitment to always contribute to the research despite the fact that she has 'a day job' as well. Her link into the university is really vital and we are more than lucky to have this connection and her incredible commitment. This core of three people do most of the hands-on work, keeping everything linked together and maintaining a focus on both the specific research activity of the day as well as the wider research program of which each project must be a part. We also have three team members who bring differing perspectives in terms of culture, gender, community, end user, and who also from time to time undertake specific research tasks, such as interviewing, running focus groups, assisting with recruitment of participants, analysis and so on. These other team members . . . have a clear and significant contribution to make in terms of supporting us in the daily work, bringing a range of perspectives to planning data collection, analysis and other activities and to ensuring that we keep the focus on the bigger picture. This seems to work well and provide people with a place to make a really valuable contribution to the ongoing development of the research without having to feel that they need to 'go out there and do some research' or they have not contributed.

Dorothy: Your study involved some particularly complex and interrelated ethical and organisational issues. Can you say something about these issues and the processes you developed for addressing them?

Robyn: We obtained ethics approval early on and have reviewed ethical procedures as necessary. If our research caused problems for the agency and became intrusive we reviewed this and changed our practice, for example, the timing of interviews.

Jackie: The ethical issues related to the range of consents that were required and what happened, for instance, if a worker did not want to participate but a client did or vice versa. There were some related issues around the way that some of the qualitative research strategies could 'mimic' early intervention work because of the emphasis upon building a relationship with participants and talking through the issues that brought them to the agency in the first place. We did not anticipate this issue, although once it happened, it seemed so obvious. In both of these situations, we used a fairly standard approach to problem resolution—being available to talk issues through until all parties were happy that they had been resolved, and being open to modifications to research design so that new information about the impact of the research on practice could be heard and effectively responded to. I think it is important to be aware that in agency research the primary responsibility is to make sure that the intervention takes place—that the client gets the support they need and research does not have a right to undermine that.

45

So whereas in other research we may just be able to go out there and capture the information we need, in agency research we need to be able to be more responsive to the particularities of each situation we encounter and to modify our plans accordingly. Sometimes this means we get a less than ideal data capture, but that is the way it is and we do not have a right to undermine interventions in the pursuit of good quality data.

Another issue was the potential for research data to be used in staff evaluations. This was one of the reasons that lay behind the decision to set up the research centre as functionally separate from the service delivery arm of the organisation and also for building a strong relationship with the university. We maintained research records really carefully and in fact were never asked to furnish information to the organisation about performance issues. I think the organisation was very aware of this issue and handled the boundaries really well.

Our background in qualitative research helped us to deal effectively with many of these challenges because of the focus on developing and maintaining good research relationships that will sustain intense research. So our work emphasised working with people to find solutions to their concerns that could then be fitted into our methodology rather than simply telling them 'that was the way it had to be'.

Comments

It can readily be seen from the above examples of qualitative research that the researcher is indeed the instrument of their own research and that the interpersonal relationships and dynamics which can emerge are complex and deeply charged for both the researcher and the researched. Such research calls for researchers of the highest personal and professional integrity with a deep capacity for reflexivity.

When we listen to these direct accounts we can see how unique each study is and how guidelines for conducting ethical research can only ever be that—just guidelines. We can also see how qualitative research, particularly with people who have additional vulnerabilities, can pose serious risks to their well-being.

However, while no research is without risks, the risks must be balanced against the possible gains from conducting such research. It can be argued that it may be unethical not to do research in the human services in which the community invests scarce resources and where professional practice is itself often an untested social experiment with the potential to hurt as well as help individuals and their families. In that sense, research is an essential tool in improving services and making them more accountable. Qualitative research in particular has given groups of people previously denied a voice the opportunity to be heard for the first time. It is a powerful tool and one to be used with care.

3

In-depth interviewing

In-depth interviewing is the most commonly used data collection approach in qualitative research. This is hardly surprising, given the common concern of qualitative researchers to understand the meaning people make of their lives from their own perspective. The in-depth interview takes seriously the notion that people are experts on their own experience and so best able to report how they experienced a particular event or phenomenon. If we interview different people about the same event or phenomenon, we will inevitably get a range of perspectives. Where the research question requires it, the perspectives of members of a range of groups, such as clients and workers, or teachers, students and parents, should be obtained.

This chapter commences with discussion of the relative strengths and weaknesses of in-depth interviews as an approach to data collection. This is followed by an outline of the interview process, from selection of participants, through the initial contact, the interview itself and ending. We have also included a section on focus groups as a special type of interview situation. The latter part of the chapter includes two field stories of research that used in-depth interviews.

Choosing in-depth interviewing

Like any method of data collection, in-depth interviews have their relative strengths and weaknesses. Ultimately the choice to use them or not must be made in relation to the nature of the data sought and the practical constraints of the research context. The best data collection approach for any study is that which will yield data that best meet the research purpose and answer the research questions. Sometimes interviews will be most appropriate, sometimes observation or the analysis of existing records. These are unlikely to be all-or-nothing questions, though. In many cases, a combination of approaches will be indicated—to answer different parts of the research question, or to provide an alternative data source that may serve to strengthen the overall findings. Very often the researcher will have to weigh up the pros and cons of a number of approaches and make the best choice available in the circumstances.

In-depth interviews do, however, have particular strengths. First, they share the general advantages of face-to-face interviewing. Their immediacy and relational quality afford considerable flexibility to the data collection process, both in terms of areas explored and the direction of the discussion. On this point, Brenner, Brown and Canter say:

> Probably the central value of the interview as a research procedure is that it allows *both* parties to explore the meaning of the questions and answers involved. There is an implicit, or explicit sharing and/or negotiation of understanding in the interview situation which is not so central, and often not present, in other research procedures. Any misunderstandings on the part of the interviewer or the interviewee can be checked immediately in a way that is just not possible when questionnaires are being completed, or tests are being performed (Brenner, Brown & Canter, 1985, p. 3).

The advantage of being able to clarify what the other means, there and then, is arguably more apparent the less structured and more conversational the interview process.

Holstein and Gubrium talk of interviewing as an active, meaning-making process.

> Both parties to the interview are necessarily and ineluctably *active*. Meaning is not merely elicited by apt questioning, nor simply transported through respondent replies; it is actively and communicatively assembled in the interview encounter. Respondents are not so much repositories of knowledge—treasuries of information awaiting excavation, so to speak—as they are constructors of knowledge in collaboration with interviewers (Holstein & Gubrium, 1997, p. 114).

Viewing interviews in this way requires attention to the interview process and context as well as the content of what is said, to the hows as well as the whats. Nevertheless, Holstein and Gubrium caution against being so concerned with interview process that what is actually said is lost.

> While the emphasis on process has sharpened concern with, and debate over, the epistemological status of interview data, it is important not to lose track of *what* is being asked about in interviews and, in turn, *what* is being conveyed by respondents. A narrow focus on *how* tends to displace the significant *whats*—the meanings—that serve as the relevant grounds for asking and answering questions (1997, p. 115).

In-depth interviews are particularly useful when the phenomena under investigation cannot be observed directly (Taylor & Bogdan, 1998). Thus they are an excellent means of finding out how people think or feel in relation to a given topic. They also enable us to talk with people about events that happened in the past and those that are yet to happen. These retrospective and anticipatory elements open up a world of experience that is not accessible via methods such as observation. Other than through diaries or other records made at the time, interviews in the present are the only way to access a person's perceptions of past events. Even then, we are as reliant on what the reporter chose to write down at the time as we are on what interview respondents choose to tell us.

It is important not to let this ability to talk with others about past experiences lead to a false sense of access to the past. The only perspective that can be obtained is that of the present, no matter that the events, thoughts and feelings being reported have already occurred. We can find out how someone feels now about what happened in the past, even what they say now about how they felt then, but this does not give us access to the past. Interviews also happen at a cross-section in time and, just as events have inevitably been reconstructed at the time of the interview, further reconstructions are undoubtedly to come. Participants' perspectives can only be presented in the context of lives as they are being lived (Langness & Frank, 1981). The process of telling their stories about the past in the present, and particularly in the interview context, will itself impact on participants' subsequent organisation and understanding of their experience (Kleinman, 1988). As Bruner states:

Stories give meaning to the present and enable us to see that present as a set of relationships involving a constituted past and a future. But narratives change, all stories are partial, all meanings incomplete. There is no fixed meaning in the past, for with each new telling the context varies, the audience differs, the story is modified . . . (Bruner, 1986, p. 153).

There are other reasons to be cautious when using in-depth interviews. No matter how much we try to construct the research process so that participants control its process, there is always power inherent in the researcher role. Ribbens expresses concern about this issue, particularly in relation to the vulnerability of research participants vis-à-vis the researcher.

The particular paradox that is worrying about depth interviews is that you give the interviewee the power to control the interview itself, and yet as a result they put themselves very much in your hands by exposing themselves in a one-sided relationship. When you come to depart you take their words away, to be objectified in an interview transcript. In the end you are very powerful in this style of interviewing, and the absence of the questionnaire may obscure this all the more (see Finch, 1984; and Stacey, 1988 on this point) (Ribbens, 1989, p. 587).

Finally, interviews allow access to what people say but not to what they do. The only way to find out what 'actually happens' in a given situation is through observation (Chapter 4).

The interview process

In-depth interviewing in qualitative research involves much more than the actual interview interaction. We now consider the stages involved in setting up and conducting in-depth interviews, from the selection of participants through to the ending of the interview encounter. Each of these stages is important and will have an impact, for better or worse, on how research participants experience the research process and on the overall quality of the research.

Finding and selecting participants

Experience of the topic under investigation and articulateness are commonly regarded as essential criteria for the inclusion of participants in qualitative research projects (Collaizzi, 1978; Wertz & van Zuuren, 1987; Polkinghorne, 1989). With specific reference to phenomenological research, Polkinghorne sees it as a requirement that research participants have 'the capacity to provide full and sensitive descriptions of the experience under investigation' (1989, p. 47). For Wertz and van Zuuren, participants need to have or be able to 'develop some significant relationship with the phenomenon under study' (1987, p. 11).

If this condition were present in every participant, we would have the 'dream team' of research participants. This is, of course, not always possible. In Chapter 5 we talk with Tim and Wendy Booth about their approach to interviewing people with an intellectual disability, people who, while certainly having experience of the research topic, have limited capacity to report it articulately.

There is no easy answer to the question as to how many participants are required for a qualitative study. It really does depend on the study. Generally speaking, there will be both theoretical and practical considerations. Theoretically, optimal numbers will be determined by the research topic and question—what you are wanting to find out, from whom, and the likely variability of experience of the phenomenon under investigation.

Theoretical sampling (Glaser & Strauss, 1967; Strauss & Corbin, 1990, 1998) is a useful approach to selecting participants, whether or not all the stages of grounded theory are being used in a particular study. In theoretical sampling, the researcher engages in a cyclical process of data collection, analysis and further data collection. After the first few interviews, further participants are sought specifically for their capacity to help fill gaps in the data that are thrown up in analysis.

Covering the range of experiences involves deliberately seeking out people whose situations and experiences are different from those already obtained, in order to obtain the broadest possible reach of the range of perspectives on the topic under investigation. The process is sometimes referred to as negative case analysis (Strauss & Corbin, 1990; Morse, 1994). Such cases 'don't necessarily negate our questions or statements, or disprove them, rather they add variation and depth of understanding' (Strauss & Corbin, 1990, p. 109, bold in original). Later in this chapter, Angelina Yuen-Tsang talks in some detail about how she used a similar process to obtain the participants for her study.

As a general rule, the relative diversity or homogeneity of

experience of the topic will impact on how many participants are needed. Where there are many possible experiences of a phenomenon, it will be important to talk to people representing a wide range of views and situations to build up a broad understanding of the topic. Even so, in situations where there is relative homogeneity, it would be wise to obtain the maximum number of participants possible in order to document the extent of the views or situations identified and to avoid the charge of choosing only the few cases that fitted the researcher's own perspective.

While each person's experience and perspective will be different, and there is always something new to hear, data collection has to stop somewhere. Where new broad patterns do not appear to be emerging, where interviewees' perspectives are confirmatory rather than contradictory, it can be safe to stop. In most cases it will not be possible to decide theoretically at the beginning just how many participants will be needed.

Qualitative research is, however, labour intensive and time consuming, from data collection through to analysis, so there will often be practical constraints on the number of people who can be interviewed. Some of the 'it depends' issues here relate to the number of study groups, the number of methods and the number of interviews. If, for example, it is important to a study to interview a number of players—as in Trinder, Beek and Connolly's (2001) study of mothers', fathers' and children's experiences of post-divorce contact, or Darlington and Bland's (1999) study of client, family and worker experiences of hope in relation to mental illness—it would be wise to limit the number of each group. Similarly, if a combination of methods is to be used, say observation, document analysis and interviews, or if multiple interviews are to be conducted with each participant, this will limit the total number of participants possible relative to available research resources.

Experienced researchers will know, however, that potential research participants are not always easy to find. Participation in qualitative research requires a considerable commitment of time and energy and, often, the willingness to commit to reflection on deeply personal experiences. Researchers often have to take as many participants as they can get, within the constraints of time and other resources. It is common to have to try a number of avenues, each with its own pros and cons. Above all, leave plenty of time for data collection and have something else to do (for example, literature review, beginning analysis) while building up the numbers. If obtaining numbers turns out not to be an issue, then the theoretical considerations can take precedence. In reality, the ability to pick and choose respondents on theoretical grounds is a luxury we have rarely encountered.

Making a connection (establishing rapport)

The development of trust between researcher and participant is an essential part of the research process. Participation in a research project about personal, and perhaps traumatic, experiences requires a great deal of trust—trust that the researcher will listen, will treat participants fairly, will respect their limits about what they want to say, and will deal with the data fairly. Without some sense of connection, of relationship, respondents are unlikely to be either sufficiently relaxed to enter into thorough exploration of the issues under discussion, or trusting enough to share their thoughts with the interviewer.

Rapport is often included in research texts as an entity that is established at the beginning of the research, and once this is done the researcher can get on with the business of researching. But rapport is not a finite commodity that can be turned on and off by the researcher. It is relational. It develops, or does not, between the researcher and the research participant. It is not 'established' once and for all. Like all relationships, the researcher–participant relationship is subject to continuing negotiation and reworking; this extends to the participant's trust in the researcher's behaviour and integrity at every stage of the research. For the researcher, it requires that they be genuinely interested in the issue being researched and in the participant's experience of it, and that they be able to communicate this interest and concern to the participant.

There are times when a strong connection between the researcher and participant can, if the researcher is not careful, impede the data collection process. As a sense of shared understanding develops, participants may take it for granted that the interviewer understands what they are talking about and skip over important aspects of their story. We really do want to know exactly what participants think about a situation and at times we want them to state the obvious—if the participant didn't say it, we can't use it as data, no matter how deep the sense of shared understanding between interviewer and interviewee. It could be reported as the interviewer's experience but not as that of the interviewee.

There is a related risk that the interviewer will think they know what the participant means and impose assumptions on the data without checking them out with participants. This can especially be an issue in 'insider' research, where researchers may assume shared understandings between themselves and the participants. Similarly, participants may be constrained and potentially self-censor what they say as a result of presumed, but mistaken or incomplete, shared understandings between them and the researcher. Miller and Glassner (1997) suggest that too close an identification with one position in relation to the social phenomenon being investigated may restrict 'which cultural stories interviewees may tell and how these may be told' (1997, p. 104).

To enable people to tell their stories, in their way, there needs to be an openness to whatever perspective may emerge. Where differences between the researcher and those being interviewed are such that rapport may not be easily established—differences of race, ethnicity, age, gender, disability, dress or language—and where resources allow, it is well worth employing interviewers who share more of the characteristics of the study group than the researcher. In her study of the experiences, attitudes and values of street-frequenting young people of non-English speaking background in Sydney, Pe-Pua (1996) hired bilingual interviewers from among street workers, youth workers and street-frequenting young people and used them to recruit as well as interview young people.

The initial contact

Prior to meeting the researcher, prospective participants have presumably been sufficiently interested to respond to information they have received about a study, but have not yet consented to participate. The initial contact (we prefer a face-to-face meeting) is their opportunity to find out more about the study, to ask any questions they may have and, most importantly, to meet the person with whom they are being asked to talk about themselves. If interviews are to be taped, it is important that permission is obtained at this stage. Once discussion about the research process is exhausted, and the prospective participant indicates they would like to proceed, they can then be asked to sign a formal consent form. Ideally, this meeting will take place on a separate day to the interview as this gives the participant time to follow-up any further questions that may arise for them and also allows a cooling off period, in which they may still change their mind about participating in the study.

Where the research topic has the potential to be distressing for the participant, it is important to work out a plan to deal with such distress should it arise. An immediate issue is to be clear about the participant's right to terminate the interview at any time. Often human research ethics committees will require that provision be made for referral to a trained professional should participants become distressed or disturbed during the course of the research. This is relatively straightforward where participants have been recruited through a professional agency. At other times it may be necessary for the researcher to set up an arrangement with an agency for referral. This should always be discussed with partici-pants, in order to work out a process for this to happen. For example, under what circumstances might referral occur—would it be self-referral only or would there be circumstances in which the researcher might make a referral on behalf of the participant? The decisions made will depend very much on the research topic, on whether appropriate resources are readily available and on the capacity of participants to access them, as well as the vulnerability of the participant group and the wishes of individual participants.

The interview

While interviews do vary in terms of how focused they are and the extent to which participants are encouraged to 'direct' the flow of the conversation, the idea of an 'unstructured' interview is really a myth. Every interview, no matter how free flowing in terms of topics and the order in which they are covered, has a structure of some sort. The interview itself is a structured social interaction—the very act of setting it up brings its own structure and context. There would be little point in conducting an interview if the interviewer did not have some idea of why they wanted to talk with that person and of what they would like to talk about. On the other hand, if the researcher imposes too much structure, many of the advantages of the in-depth interview will be diminished. There is a fine line between having enough structure to facilitate talk (why are we here?) and imposing a structure that becomes constraining for the participant. The extent to which interviews are focused depends on many things, including the purpose of the study, the nature of the data sought, and pragmatic concerns about time and other resources.

In most cases an interview guide is recommended. This could be as simple as a list of topics to be covered during the interview. It does not necessarily commit the interviewer to covering those topics in any particular order.

Effective in-depth interviewing requires considerable skill, and people with formal training and experience in communication and counselling skills start with something of an advantage. While there are similarities in the communication skills used in research interviewing and clinical interviewing, the purposes of the two forms are, however, different and should not be confused. It is important that interviewers understand their role as researcher and do not slip into counselling mode. Research interviewing can certainly have therapeutic effects, but it may be precisely because it is not therapy that this is possible. Research interviews carry no expectation that the interviewee will change their lives—we are, after all, interested in them as they are. In-depth interviews may also be longer and less focused than interviews in therapy contexts. Paradoxically, this may afford interviewees a greater capacity to explore their experiences than is possible in some therapy contexts. One participant in Yvonne Darlington's sexual abuse study said:

> In the interview I could almost at times just see myself again and actually talking about things, I was feeling that little girl again . . . and that has not happened to me. I've had some memories but no feelings. To get the two together was a new experience . . . I think maybe I just let go of something . . . I've been in counselling and I've been in support groups where a lot of this does get talked about and I've never had that same feeling. So I'd say it would be the fact that it was an interview . . . I definitely didn't feel under pressure here but sometimes in counselling or support group I feel under pressure so I tend to get defensive and back off (Darlington, 1993, p. 111).

In any interview, different types of questions will elicit different types of responses. Descriptive questions about what and how things happened are particularly useful in encouraging people to describe their experiences. 'Why' questions, on the other hand, may seem interrogatory and can lead to dead ends. Interestingly, 'what' and 'how' sometimes implicitly contain elements of 'why'. They are not only less likely to be experienced as intrusive but may yield explanations anyway. On this point, Becker says:

Somehow 'Why?' seems more profound, more intellectual, as though you were asking about the deeper meaning of things, as opposed to the simple narrative 'How?' would likely evoke . . . 'How?' questions, when I asked them, gave people more leeway, were less constraining, invited them to answer in any way that suited them, to tell a story that included whatever they thought the story ought to include in order to make sense. They didn't demand a 'right' answer, didn't seem to be trying to place responsibility for bad actions or outcomes anywhere (Becker, 1998, pp. 58–9).

Clarificatory questions are also useful. If a word or concept is unfamiliar to the researcher, a simple, 'When you say . . . I'm not exactly sure what you mean. Could you tell me a little more about that?' can provide the necessary clarification and open up further exploration.

Some studies require attention to subtle nuances of questioning in order to elicit the type of material sought. Where the focus is on descriptions of experience rather than descriptions of objects and actions, as is often the case in interpretive studies, questions such as 'What did you experience?' and 'What was it like for you?' are more likely to elicit experiential data than questions such as 'What happened?' (Polkinghorne, 1989, p. 46).

Tomm's (1988) typology of lineal, circular, strategic and reflexive questions was developed for a therapeutic context but also has applicability to research interviewing. The types can be seen as reflecting two main types of interviewer intent: orienting (lineal, circular) and influencing (strategic, reflexive). Lineal questions include all the what, where, how and why questions that are commonly used in research contexts and are primarily investigative in intent. Circular questions are more exploratory in their intent, and as such can be useful in opening up discussion of people's perceptions of a complex event or phenomenon, including their thoughts on how others might see the situation. They are less useful in eliciting direct narratives (What happened next?). The idea of using 'influencing' questions seems anathema in social research, and we cannot think of a place for Tomm's strategic questions, which are leading, directive and have a corrective intent. Reflexive questions, while also influencing, are facilitative in intent and can be useful in opening up discussion of hypothetical situations, the 'what do you think would happen if' and 'can you imagine' questions that may facilitate talk about future hopes and expectations.

Most researchers go into in-depth interviews with some kind of interview guide or list of topics to cover at some stage during the interview. This can serve as a useful reminder of core aspects of the research question to be asked about. While there are no hard and fast rules as to what should be in an interview guide, less is generally best. Too much detail will be difficult to read and will distract the interviewer's attention from what the interviewee is saying. Any attempt to rigidly follow a guide in a set order will inevitably interrupt the conversational flow and cut across the aim of encouraging participants to talk about what is of concern to them, in the way that best facilitates that. As Burgess (1984) found in his interviews with schoolchildren, different people's stories unfold in different ways and what may seem a logical order to one person may be quite inhibiting for another.

Recording

In-depth interviews should, if at all possible, be taped. Even if it were possible to take notes at the speed that the interview progressed, this would be very distracting for the interviewee and also make it virtually impossible for the interviewer to attend to the crucial relational aspects of the interview. It goes without saying that a good quality tape recorder is essential. While in practice many interviewees become used to the presence of a tape recorder quite readily, it makes sense to use equipment that is least likely to cause distraction. Smaller is generally better, preferably with a built-in microphone. Grbich (1999) suggests a roving microphone for interviews where you are likely to have to move around, for example when interviewing children. For interviews with more than one person, a flat microphone on a table works well. For focus groups, two tape recorders may ease anxiety about picking up everything that is said. Transcribe from one, using the other for backup when something can't be heard properly. Always use new batteries and always take spares.

Tape quality is always a concern in qualitative research. While good quality equipment will take you part of the way, there are more considerations to naturalistic research than finding the optimum taping conditions. Interviews are often conducted in people's homes where there are distractions that may not be able to be controlled—children playing, television in another room, the neighbour mowing the lawn, a busy road outside, being under a flight path—these day-to-day noises do not stop just because we want to interview someone. The interview content itself can impact on tape quality—people's voices may fade if they become distressed. There will be times when the only option is to pause the tape. While it is helpful to discuss at the initial contact the importance of relative quiet and uninterrupted time, we need to be careful not to cross that bridge where we seem to be dictating to our research participants how they should be in their own homes.

Ending

Every social interaction has a beginning, a middle and an end, and for the interaction to be completed successfully, in a manner satisfactory to all parties, each part has to go well. Research interactions are no exception.

In considering endings, we need to think of the ending of each interaction, if there are to be multiple interviews, as well as the ending of the participant's involvement in the research.

There will always be obligations to report back to participants at some stage—being given a copy of a research report or information on how to access it would be minimal. Further ongoing contact may well have been negotiated. The important thing is that both researcher and participant are clear about what is expected and that the researcher both follows through on mutually agreed arrangements and does not create expectations of ongoing involvement that they are not able or prepared to meet.

The ending of each interaction is no less important and needs to be planned for. Endings should not come as a surprise. Being clear about the time each has available to talk at the beginning of the interview establishes the parameters of the interaction. Even so, it is generally helpful to include some reminders towards the latter part of the interview, particularly if the participant has become very involved in talking about their experiences and the conversation seems not to be coming to a natural end. Such reminders should be given in plenty of time, not just five minutes before the end of the interview. It can be helpful to let the participant know where you are in the process, for example, 'I have just a couple more things I'd like to ask you about'. Always ask whether there is anything else they would like to say—and leave time for them to say it. Also consider that you may need to leave time to negotiate another contact if an interview is unexpectedly long and time is running out.

Generally, the more intense the interaction, the more time people will need to wind down emotionally. Always leave time for some day-to-day conversation at the end of the interview—some people will not want to engage at this level but for others it will be an important part of the closure process. It shows you have a genuine interest in them as a person and not just a research topic. Saying yes to a cup of tea that is offered can be an important message of acceptance of the interviewee as a person. It is unlikely to signal the opening of the floodgates of never-ending contact, as some researchers may fear. It is more likely to provide the time and space for a real and meaningful interaction that enables both researcher and participant to effectively disengage from the relationship. Remember that in many cases people achieve a level of sharing and disclosure about themselves in in-depth interviews that is rare in everyday life; it is important that they feel they have been dealt with sensitively and are not left feeling emotionally raw or used.

Sometimes the researcher will need some assistance to work through emotions aroused during interviews. In the case of research on topics that are potentially disturbing, it is important to have a debriefing strategy worked out beforehand. Writing down your reactions can be a valuable aid to debriefing, as can talking with a supervisor or trusted colleague, but be careful not to jeopardise confidentiality.

Focus groups

Long used in market research, focus groups have been increasingly used in social science research since the 1980s. This is still a developing area and the trend is towards expansion of the possibilities for their use rather than narrowly prescribing how and when they should be used (Morgan 1997). Like interviews, focus groups vary on a continuum from highly structured through to relatively unstructured and data obtained from focus groups can be analysed quantitatively or qualitatively.

Focus groups share many of the advantages of in-depth interviews as a means of data collection. Basch says, for example, that 'Focus group interviews are particularly well suited to collecting in-depth, qualitative data about individuals' definitions of problems, opinions and feelings, and meanings associated with various phenomena' (1987, p. 434).

Particular advantages of focus groups relate to the benefits of group interaction, such as the extent to which the cross-flow of communication sparks ideas that would not emerge as easily in a one-to-one interview. Groups also take the pressure off participants to respond to every question. Hearing others talk about their experiences, in a supportive environment, may enable participants to feel comfortable about sharing their own experiences. The group context also enables exploration of a range of subjective responses in relation to one or more topics in a relatively short space of time and relatively economically (Basch, 1987; Mariampolski, 1989; Morgan, 1997).

It is also in relation to the group interaction that potential disadvantages of focus groups arise. These relate to the extent to which participants may experience peer pressure to remain silent about some views or to readily agree with more dominant views in the group. With sensitive topics there is the potential for embarrassment, and participants may be reluctant to talk about personal experiences. Focus groups also place limits on the amount of time each participant has to speak. In-depth interviews allow for concentrated and uninterrupted focus on the perceptions of one person and are preferred when this is sought.

As with any qualitative research, participants in focus groups should be given as much information as possible about the purpose of the research and the topics to be discussed and given the opportunity to opt out if they do not feel able to participate comfortably in group discussion. It is in the initial pre-group meeting that trust begins to be established. Issues of trust apply to focus groups as much as they do to in-depth interviews. Unless there is trust in the facilitator—that they will be heard when they speak, their contribution will be valued, they will not be pressured to speak when they don't want to or about things they don't want to talk about, and that they will be 'protected' from the group if needs be—prospective participants are not likely to agree to take part. Worse, they may choose to participate and, if their trust turns out to be unwarranted, be at emotional risk in the process.

Darlington, Osmond and Peile (2001) used focus groups in a study of child welfare workers' use of theory in practice. They were used as a third stage of data collection, following two in-depth interviews, so participants had developed considerable trust in the researchers by this stage. The focus groups involved two activities. The first activity involved presenting back to participants the thematic analysis of the material obtained from two rounds of in-depth interviews in order to check the validity of interpretations made. We followed this with a theory representation exercise that examined how participants utilised theory in practice. Participants were requested to portray diagrammatically their perceptions of how they integrated physical abuse theory in their practice and then to explain their drawing to the group. We were impressed by their willingness to discuss their practice in the group and so risk exposure. We attributed this to the trust that had developed between participants and researchers and the commonality of work-setting shared by participants—although the latter could have led to competition and defensiveness among participants had trust not been present.

As with in-depth interviews, attention needs to be paid to designing the types of questions that will be most effective in eliciting the type of material sought. If the focus of the research is about feelings and experiences, at some stage the focus group will have to move beyond description of events in order to find out about participants' experiences of them.

For sensitive topics, Mariampolski (1989) suggests commencing with relatively 'safe' issues and encouraging everyone in the group to speak early on, only moving on to more sensitive topics when there is evidence that participants are ready to do so. Equally important is the winding down period at the end. A return to 'safe' topics is advisable, in order to reach some closure to the discussion of potentially stressful subjects.

Stories from the field

The first story from the field is from Angelina Yuen-Tsang's study of the social support networks of working mothers in Beijing, the second from Yvonne's study of women who had been sexually abused in childhood.

Angelina Yuen-Tsang—Social support networks of Chinese working mothers in Beijing

We introduced Angelina Yuen-Tsang in Chapter 2 where she talked about the process of choosing a community in which to conduct her research and her engagement with that community. The study had several stages of data collection, including focus groups, observation and in-depth interviews with 27 working mothers. Here she talks about the three stages of data collection and the process of selecting the women to interview.

Focus groups and observation

Angelina: After gaining entry to the community, I started to do some focus groups, partly because I felt that I didn't know enough about the culture in the Beijing community. I felt that I needed to know more about their way of life, their perceptions, et cetera, because most of the available literature was from overseas countries. Even though it talked a lot about social support, I didn't learn a lot about how social support is being rendered in mainland China. So I used focus groups to alert me to underlying issues that I may not be aware of. For example, I asked people about their pattern of social support, the issues they encounter and any tensions that they experience. I also asked them to comment on some concepts or ideas from the western literature. This helped me to design my question guideline, even though I didn't follow it in the end, but at least the focus groups alerted me to a lot of issues which I was not aware of earlier . . . The participant observation was also very important because I felt that, in order to understand the local community and its dynamics, I have to know the community well. So I lived in a local hotel right in the middle of the community, and I tried to observe the community at different times. For example I'd get up very early and wander around the community because the community virtually woke up at around five or six and a lot of people were going to work and so on. So I'd go out at different times of the day and try to see the pattern of their daily routine . . . I'd chat with them and see the pattern of their daily life and how they interact, how they chat, what the topics of their conversations are, what their concerns are and things like that.

Yvonne: So a lot of that was orienting you to the community, helping you to get some sense of what life was like in that community.

Angelina: And also helping me to understand the context of their lives because when I started to do the interviews, I needed to know what they were talking about and to be able to strike up a conversation. So it helped a lot.

The interviews

Angelina: I remember that for the first interview, I had a very detailed question guideline set up after the focus groups, but in the end I think I only asked a few questions from it. I then decided not to use it at all because I found that if I followed the question guideline mechanically, it ruined my relationship with the interviewee and the flow of conversation . . . so I still had a set of questions at the back of my mind but these questions were rather free-flowing and open-ended. I tried to follow [the interviewee's] direction as it went . . . for me the most important question was to find out about the flow of their life course and the most critical events they encounter. Also, during these critical events, what kind of support do they receive, from whom, and how and what kind of difficulties do they encounter—do they really receive the help that they would like to receive and what are the consequences, et cetera. In addition, I wanted to know their values and their perceptions of the whole process. So these were basically the major issues that I had. Other than that, all the little questions didn't really matter, so after the first interview I decided to scrap the guideline and just let the conversation flow.

Yvonne: And did you tape the interviews?

Angelina: Yes. I asked the interviewees' permission and usually in the beginning they were a little bit cautious but gradually they began to enjoy doing the interview.

Yvonne: Were there cultural issues around the process of interviewing? I'm wondering was this an unfamiliar kind of encounter for the women?

Angelina: I think it was something that most of them had not encountered. That's why I think some of them enjoyed the interview because they felt that they were being treated with respect. They felt that they had a chance to talk about their underlying feelings which they don't get the chance to share with other people, even with their relatives or close friends or whatever. And also [the interview] was about something they probably had not thought of before, because in their daily encounters with friends and relatives they seldom talked about support and what kind of support they receive from their relatives and what kind of impact that support has on them. They have not thought of things in this way. So I think most of them were very interested in the process because they hadn't had that sort of relationship in the past—a very, not intense, but very close interaction in which they could talk heart-to-heart with another woman about their personal feelings or their problems. A few of them have written to me afterwards saying how much they have enjoyed the interview, and one or two of them said that I've helped them even though I didn't intend to do so . . .

Yvonne: Did the women talk easily about their feelings? If this was an unusual situation for them, did it take a while for some of them to warm up?

Angelina: Oh sure, yes. It took some time to warm up but many of them revealed their feelings, even though a lot of my academic friends were rather suspicious. They said that it would not be easy to get them to reveal their feelings but I found it was not that difficult. There were a few with whom I had a very good rapport . . . but for some it was probably the local official's introduction that made them decide to be interviewed, so they regarded it as a duty or whatever . . . So there were a few who just did the interview as dutiful interviewees, but even they answered the questions and I managed to get the information that I needed.

Sampling

Yvonne: With the interviews you used theoretical sampling and you said that in some cases it took a while to find just the right person. Can you talk a little bit about how that process worked?

Angelina: I remember, say for the first ten interviews, that I asked the local officials to help me to identify people with different characteristics. So I worked out a table— I needed people from different occupations, different age groups and different family compositions, say for example a nuclear family, or three generations living together or two generations together, et cetera. So it's the age group, the occupation group, the education background, the family type and the type of residence . . . but after the first ten or so, I gradually realised that I needed more interviewees of certain types. For example, initially they gave me the better families, the families that were harmonious, reputed for their good relationships and so on. So I told them I needed some families that had problems. For example, I said, I need some who are in a worse financial situation, and some not from the state-owned factories. Those who worked in state-owned factories at that time were relatively better off in terms of their welfare. So I said I needed some from the street-level factories and some who were self-employed because at that time there were more and more self-employed persons—working the streets selling fruit, selling clothes, things like that. I also wanted some who had a difficult relationship with their in-laws or husband. So gradually I generated more and more questions . . . for example, I found that those living in three-generation families had more support. These supports are holistic and more comprehensive but there obviously are many families without that full range of support. So I needed those who were more isolated, without many relatives in Beijing . . . because I felt that there must be families that were not that well supported, and there must be families that were not that ideal, not so harmonious. If they have strained relationships with their relatives, then what happens to their support and if their support from their work organisations breaks down, which was happening at that time, then what happens? Things like that. So in the beginning it was the demographic considerations but gradually it was more the theoretical considerations that guided me.

Yvonne: Do you feel confident that at the end of the day you obtained a thorough mix of types of situation?

Angelina: Well, I don't think it can be perfect, but as far as my particular piece of research is concerned, after interviewing the 27 women I thought that the questions that I had at the particular time were answered—but of course there were many other questions that I would like to follow-up. But you can never follow-up all the questions and you have to set a boundary. So after doing the 27 interviews I felt that I had to make a stop to it, otherwise it would go on forever.

Yvonne Darlington—The experience of childhood sexual abuse

Yvonne: I talked earlier (Chapter 1) about how I became interested in this research topic and my choice of a qualitative methodology. In this chapter, I'll comment on two aspects of the interviews: my interviewing style and the women's reports of their experience of the in-depth interview, as reported during the follow-up interview. Ten women participated in the study. I had three meetings with each of them: the initial contact in which we negotiated their participation in the study, the in-depth interview and the follow-up interview. The in-depth and follow-up interviews were both taped and transcribed.

Interviewing style

The in-depth interviews were relatively unstructured. I had a short list of topics to cover but imposed no constraints on the women in terms of the order in which topics were covered or how much they talked about each. Even so, we both knew that the expectation was that they would talk about their experience of sexual abuse, so the research was constructed in such a way that child sexual abuse was brought into focus. Nevertheless, I encouraged the women to talk about those aspects of their lives that they considered relevant to the study rather than just the sexual abuse. This approach seems to have worked to the extent that the women did talk about other aspects of their lives and some in fact volunteered that other sorts of abuse, such as verbal abuse and putdowns in childhood, had had a more lasting impact on their sense of self than the sexual abuse.

Given the focus on the women's stories, as they wished to tell them, I chose a deliberately reflective style of interviewing. As far as was possible, my questions flowed from or built upon a woman's previous comments. They were often clarificatory in nature. Sometimes I asked questions that led women to state what was, in the context of our discussion, obvious. There were times when an appropriate therapeutic response would have been an empathic nod. In the research context, I asked the naive questions so participants could actually state what was implicit, but unspoken.

Except when clarification was needed, I took the approach of letting the women talk until they had exhausted what they had to say on a particular topic. There were times when what a woman was saying did not seem, to me, to be immediately relevant to her experience of sexual abuse. At these times, I resisted the temptation to cut in and inevitably the connections the woman was making between the various aspects of her life story became clear. There were other times when the women's comments related directly to things I wanted to explore further. While I did not want to break their train of thought and thus risk 'losing' what they were about to say, neither did I want to 'lose' the new avenue for discussion. I managed this by jotting down brief notes, no more than a word or two, about leads to follow-up later. More often than not, the woman came to the point I had jotted down herself later in the interview. It was only towards the end of the interviews that I clarified any remaining points.

Not curtailing the flow of what the women had to say also involved respecting their silences. The women differed considerably in the time they took to collect their thoughts. I needed to be sensitive to when a silence was a working silence and when it indicated the exhaustion of a topic area. I decided to err on the side of not rushing in and always checked that there was no more to be said in one area before moving to another.

There were undoubtedly many things I could have done differently. Others listening to the tapes or reading the transcripts might wonder at directions taken and things said or unsaid. One of the reasons for conducting the follow-up interviews was my curiosity about how the women had experienced the interviews. I did not expect, nor [did I] get, a detailed critique of my style, but in talking about how they experienced the interviews at follow-up, there was some validation for overall choices I had made.

The follow-up interviews

During the follow-up interview, the women talked about their experience of being interviewed and how they felt afterwards, as well as anything else they had thought of that they would like to add.

I now turn to two aspects of what the women said during the follow-up interviews that reflect methodological choices that I had made. These are: my decision to limit my contact with the women to the initial meeting and two interviews; and the decision to only include women who were referred through support groups and counsellors. Both these decisions reflected my concern for the women's well-being, that participation in the study would not prove to be detrimental to their emotional health and that, should distressing issues arise, they would already be linked to a trusted support network.

Limiting contact

My choice to contain the women's involvement in the research process rather than have it ongoing and open-ended was an attempt to minimise any potential emotional distress that the women might experience through participation in the study and to provide a clear boundary around any expectation that they talk about their experience of childhood sexual abuse in this context. This was somewhat at odds with prevailing feminist research approaches. Certainly some feminist researchers at that time encouraged multiple interviews and ongoing engagement with participants as research collaborators as ways of minimising the power differences between researcher and researched and highlighting their shared experiences as women (Oakley, 1981; Stanley & Wise, 1983; Harding, 1986). Comments by two of the women indicated that they valued the containment offered by this approach. Cynthia (all names have been changed) said at follow-up that it was the absence of an emotional tie between herself and me that enabled her to share her experiences. She contrasted her relationship with me to that of her family and friends:

> I don't feel that I'm vulnerable to you because we are not emotionally linked. I feel that you are doing a job. I'm participating in this of my own free will so I don't look at you as a threat to my innermost feelings (Darlington, 1993, p. 109).

Judith welcomed the follow-up interview as a chance to achieve closure:

> Even this morning when they asked me where I was going I said, 'I've got the follow-up interview with the researcher', and I even felt then that it was very necessary that I was going to follow it up. I felt it was good that I was going to do the follow-up—not sort of left up in the air (Darlington, 1993, p. 109).

Her comments at the end of the follow-up interview indicated that it had been a useful process for her:

> I feel much happier. I've read a few books on women's stories and that and I was thinking that's how it must feel when they've written the book. An excited feeling. Powerful . . . I'll probably go and do a little skip up the street. That's the feeling. Compared to feeling really vulnerable after the interview (Darlington, 1993, p. 109).

Referral source

My decision to include only women referred through counsellors and support groups also related to my concern that women should be readily able to obtain support in relation to any issues engendered by their participation in the research. It also enabled me to concentrate fully on my role as researcher, taking responsibility for how I related to the women as researcher but without having to cross over to a counselling role for which, in this context, I had no mandate. Two themes in the women's comments supported this decision. First, several of the women commented that participation in the study would have been difficult for them had they not already had counselling in relation to their sexual abuse, and second, even in this group of self-selected women, over two-thirds reported some degree of emotional distress following the interview.

In relation to the timing of the interview, some of the women identified a time when they would either not have made themselves available to be interviewed about their experience of sexual abuse or, if they had, would have found it emotionally detrimental. Cynthia said it had only been since she had come to believe that the sexual abuse was not her fault that she had been able to talk about it; but prior to that, she would have felt too ashamed to do an interview like this. Irene thought that, even six months earlier, she would have coped poorly with the stress of talking about such painful issues, saying, 'It could have really taken me down.' Judith would not previously have been able to participate in research on this topic as it had only been her recent recall of her sexual abuse that made her experience accessible even to herself.

Of the women who reported some degree of emotional distress following the interview, some had had regular counselling appointments or support group meetings following the interview that had helped. Others said their distress had subsided of its own accord. Nevertheless, all the women reported that they were pleased they had done the interview. Some, like Judith, found the process itself helpful:

> I can't believe it. I've actually talked nearly three hours . . . It's like I've never been able to do that before . . . but it's like that I've been allowed to say, to go on and on for nearly three hours and it's just been okay to do that. And what I was saying, maybe it was worth putting on tape (Darlington, 1996, p. 130).

Comments

In this chapter, we have seen that in-depth interviewing involves much more than what happens in the interview itself, crucial as this is. We have considered the selection of participants, the initial contact, the ending of each contact, reporting back to participants and, finally, reaching closure. Underlying all of these stages is the relationship between researcher and participant. The researcher's handling of the interaction and the extent to which they develop a trusting working relationship with their participants will always impact on the nature of the data obtained and, in many cases, has implications for the well-being of the participants. This is particularly so when the research concerns sensitive issues, as it did in both of the stories included in this chapter.

We also considered the advantages of in-depth interviews as a data collection method. These include their high degree of interactivity and capacity for responsiveness to the research context, and the capacity to obtain information about things that cannot otherwise be observed, including thoughts and emotions as well as past and future events. In the following chapter, on observation, we consider a form of data collection that can do what interviews cannot, that is, to allow us to stand aside from events and watch them as they occur.

4

Observation

Observation is a very effective way of finding out what people do in particular contexts, the routines and interactional patterns of their everyday lives. In the human services, observational research methods can provide an understanding of what is happening in the encounter between a service provider and user, or within a family, a committee, a ward or residential unit, a large organisation or a community.

Observation has a long history in ethnographic fieldwork in anthropology (Spradley, 1980) and sociology (Johnson, 1975; Hammersley & Atkinson, 1995). The many classic studies using ethnographic methods include Liebow's studies of African American street corner men (1967) and homeless women (1993), Dalton's (1959) study of formal and informal aspects of the world of managers, and Becker et al.'s (1961) study of the professional enculturation of medical students.

This chapter commences with a brief introduction to some of the practicalities of observation in human services research. We consider some of the strengths and limitations of observation, approaches to combining observation with other data collection methods, observation roles, the timing and duration of observation sessions, and recording observations. The second part of the chapter includes two edited interviews with researchers who used observation as part of their research.

Choosing observation

Like all data collection methods, observation has its strengths and limitations. In reality, every method involves trade-offs between relative strengths and relative limitations. Fortunately, we are rarely confined to just one way of collecting data. Unlike interviews and document analysis, observation affords access to events as they happen. Observation also generally requires little active effort on the part of those being observed. Unlike interviews, which can be time consuming for participants, taking not only the time for the interview but also effort in making arrangements to clear other activities, observation takes place at the same time as an activity that would be happening anyway.

The observer is, however, limited to observable social phenomena. Internal processes of cognition and emotion cannot be observed, even if non-verbal indicators of what these may be are evident. Observation alone cannot tell us why people do the things they do or what the particular activity means to them—even astute observation of non-verbal behaviour cannot provide access to a person's own understanding of why they are smiling, frowning or crying. And while observation can assist in understanding events as they unfold, events that have already occurred or that have not yet happened cannot be observed.

It is sometimes assumed that observation is more 'objective' than interviewing, because the setting is not so controlled by the researcher. Unlike the interviewer, who is intricately involved in the interaction, the observer watches what happens between others. The presence of the observer will, however, inevitably impact on the setting to varying degrees. People who know they are being watched may alter their behaviour in all sorts of ways, both consciously and unconsciously.

The observer also controls what is recorded and thus brought to analysis. Just as the information obtained from in-depth interviews reflects the interviewing style and skill of the interviewer, material obtained through observation is filtered through the observer. The observer has first to see something and then to identify it as interesting and worth reporting. Different observers undoubtedly notice different things. The research purpose, the researcher's conceptual framework and whatever other biases and assumptions they bring to the research will all influence what is noticed and what sense is made of it. These are the realities of research practice. There is always the risk of imposing one's own interpretations and assumptions on what is observed and so failing to understand what an activity means for those involved in it.

It is important to build in safeguards to minimise such misinterpretation. Understanding of the context being observed is one approach. This can be achieved either through prior familiarity with the setting or through a period of general observation at the commencement of a study. Where practicable, the use of co-observers may provide a check on observation. Are all observers seeing similar things and making similar sense of them? Where it is possible that co-observers are operating with similar biases, and that agreement reflects their shared understandings rather than what is happening in the observation setting, it may be helpful to include a naive observer, someone whose mindset is outside that of the researcher. Ultimately, there may be no better approach than checking out with the research participants themselves what their activity means to them, either in formal interviews as a further stage of data collection, or taking successive stages of analysis back to them for verification.

Combining observation with interviews

Observation can be used at different stages of a study and for different reasons. Used in the early stages of a study, it can be a useful way of understanding the context of the phenomenon under investigation and working out what the important questions to be asked are. This is particularly valuable where the researcher is unfamiliar with the phenomenon. This type of observation could precede a more structured phase of observation or other data collection methods. Later in this chapter, Anne Coleman talks about how she used observation as a basis for getting to know the research context and helping to work out what issues to explore in interviews. An equally strong argument could be made for conducting interviews first, in order to work out what are the important things, from the perspective of the study group, to look for in the observations. Cheryl Tilse's study is an example of this approach.

Observation can be particularly useful where research participants have limited verbal skills. Combining interviews and observation is a common approach in research with children and with people with learning disabilities, for example, see Chapter 5.

The observation process

We now consider some of the practicalities of observation, including observation roles, the timing and duration of observation sessions, and recording.

Observation roles

Observation roles can be viewed along a continuum from complete observer through observer-as-participant to participant-as-observer to complete participant (Gold, 1958; Adler & Adler, 1987). In a similar way, Spradley (1980) identifies five levels of participation: non-participation, passive participation, moderate participation, active participation and complete participation. Traditionally, ethnographers have accepted that most levels other than that of complete observer or non-participant will involve a degree of deception. Using deception is, however, quite problematic, both ethically and for its potential impact on the researcher. (Ethical issues in relation to the importance of obtaining informed consent to participate in research were discussed in Chapter 2.) In a personal account of the experience of participant observation, Gans says:

> A final source of anxiety is the deception inherent in participant observation . . . even though [the fieldworker] seems to give of himself when he participates, he is not really doing so and, thus, deceives the people he studies. He pretends to participate emotionally when he does not; he observes even when he does not appear to be doing so, and like the formal interviewer, he asks questions with covert purposes of which his respondents are likely to be unaware. In short, psychologically, the participant observer is acting dishonestly; he is deceiving people about his feelings, and in observing when they do not know it, he *is* spying on them . . . This has two personal consequences: a pervasive feeling of guilt and, partly in compensation, a tendency to overidentify with the people being studied (Gans, 1982, p. 59).

In this chapter we are assuming fully negotiated observer roles that do not involve deception, whatever the level of participation. By this we mean being absolutely clear about one's role as a researcher and, wherever possible, ensuring that the people actually being observed (and not just official gatekeepers) are aware of the observer's presence. Even where observation is conducted from a covert place, such as behind a one-way mirror, we assume that the observer's presence has been negotiated and that those being observed are aware they are being watched.

The observer is always in some respects a participant, as their presence will always have some impact on the setting. The level of participation that is possible or appropriate will vary from one setting to another. In many general settings, the goal of 'just blending in' is more likely to be achieved through a level of everyday participation. Non-participation to the extent of avoiding basic human interactions, such as responding to greetings, would in all likelihood draw more attention to the observer's presence and potentially heighten their impact on the setting. On the other hand, participation is unlikely to be appropriate when observing highly specialised activity, such as in an operating theatre or in a child protection or psychiatric case conference. Even where the observer is qualified to participate in such an activity, they are unlikely to be able to do justice to both roles at once.

While the boundaries of the researcher's role should be negotiated and firmly established prior to commencing the observation, in reality some flexibility may develop in the role as the research progresses. The role of uninvolved observer may be more readily sustained early on in the research when the researcher is relatively unknown in the observation setting. As those being observed become more familiar with the researcher's presence, there may be invitations, even demands, to participate. In this situation we would consider the degree of role clarity established, including clarity as to whether one is primarily participant or observer at any given time, to be the primary issue, rather than the level of participation per se.

While in practice there will often be a continuum of involvement along these dimensions, being clear about where one is (or wants to be) at any point in time is invaluable in two ways. It helps the researcher monitor how things are going, and to gauge whether boundaries need to be adjusted. It can also be helpful for those who are being observed. If the researcher is clear about their purpose and role, and is consistent in this, it will be easier for participants to accept the observer in that role and let them get about the business of observing. In a paradoxical way, participants who understand why the observer is there and what they are doing may be less bothered by their presence and the observer, in turn, may be less likely to have a negative reactive impact on the setting.

When to observe and for how long?

No social setting is static. There will always be a range of activities over time, whether during a day, a week or a month, and within each activity there are likely to be peaks and slow downs of occurrence. Realistically, one cannot hope to observe every single occurrence of an activity. A sampling process thus needs to occur. The best guide to deciding when to observe will be the research purpose. It is important to be clear about what is being observed and to take a cross-section of occurrences. It makes sense to expend valuable observation time at the times when what is being observed is most likely to happen. For example, observations of parents picking up and dropping off children to and from school would need to occur at those two times of the day. Patterns may vary on different days of the week, however (there may be daily changes in patterns of children's activities, or in parents' availability to pick their children up), or throughout the year (Do parents pick up children more commonly at the start of a new term, or during inclement weather?). Whatever the research question, it is important that the observation plan be broad enough to include any significant variations in activity that may potentially alter the conclusions drawn from the research.

The duration of any period of observation needs to be carefully considered. Observation sessions certainly have to be long enough to observe the social processes that are the subject of the study—in a study of changes in client–worker interactions at various stages of counselling sessions, for example, there would be little point in leaving before a session ended. On the other hand, observation requires considerable concentration and sessions should not be so long that alertness fades, or so much has been observed that the observer forgets or lacks the energy to record or reflect on what has happened.

Recording observations

As with so many other aspects of research practice, what and how much to record depends on the purpose of the observation and how the data are to be analysed.

For quantitative analysis, highly structured recording frames may be used (Trickett, 1993; Singh et al., 1997) that enable data to be reduced as they are recorded. This can be useful for the minute

analysis of interactional processes such as the non-verbal communication between a mother and her infant. Recording for qualitative
analysis is less structured but decisions still need to be made about
how to focus the observation—this could be at a very specific or
more general level. In the stories reported below, Cheryl Tilse
focused her recording specifically on the movements and interactions of visitors to the nursing homes, while Anne Coleman was
interested in a much broader sweep of activity in Fortitude Valley.
In each case their purpose flowed from the research question, but
the intensity of observation and recording had implications for how
long each session lasted. In general, Cheryl was able to observe for
longer periods of time than Anne, who, after a couple of hours,
became 'overloaded' with things she wanted to record.

Lofland and Lofland (1995) stress the necessity of recording as
soon as possible after observing and suggest a practical process for
dealing with the often impractical task of writing copious notes
while in the field, whether through the risk of missing something
else that is important or through concern for how those being
observed will respond to one's writing. Their suggestion is to jot
down brief notes during the observation and to write these up as
full field notes after leaving the field, but always no later than the
following morning. These notes should be as faithful a recollection
of what happened as possible, and clearly distinguish between exact
quotations, paraphrasing and more general recall. These raw field
notes should be identified separately from the researcher's own
reflections and conceptual material, which themselves may range
from brief impressions to more formal analytic notes.

Stories from the field

In each of the following inside stories, observation was used in
conjunction with several other methods of data collection, although
the interview excerpts included here focus specifically on the use
of observation. We asked both Anne Coleman and Cheryl Tilse to
begin by talking about why they chose observation as a major
method of data collection, then to move on to the practicalities of
how they went about it. These two very different examples provide
some useful insights into the versatility of observation as a method
of data collection and some of the issues to consider when thinking
about using observation.

Anne Coleman—Five star motels

Anne's was a multi-method, five-phase study, each phase building on the one before. The phases were observation, followed by informal interviews with a range of people in public spaces, then in-depth interviews with homeless people, a search of documents that related to the local urban renewal process and, finally, a second phase of observation. Anne has published on ethical issues encountered during observation (McAuliffe & Coleman, 1999) and social policy implications of the study (Coleman, 1997). She is talking here about her use of observation as a data collection method.

Choosing observation

Yvonne: Why did you choose observation as an approach to data collection?

Anne: Simply because I'd known people in this group long enough to know that in fact they could be quite devilish . . . They could, just for the fun of it, tell you the biggest story and then tell you something else the next day and then you were caught in that terrible dilemma about, well, what am I going to believe? It's also a very divided community so if you talk to one person they will tell you this is a fact and there's no question about that and if you talk to somebody else they'll tell you something else is a fact. And you find out that none of those things are actually facts . . . So I knew that observation was going to be a really useful way to check what was said to me against what I'd actually seen myself . . .

The other really important reason for doing the observation first up was that because of [my] familiarity [with the area] I had a fair degree of knowledge but I knew that some of that knowledge would be outdated . . . I wanted to go back and just have a look at the whole place and the range of things that happened in those spaces before I actually started to focus myself in again . . .

Yvonne: What were the benefits of that first stage of observation?

81

Anne: Well, the first one was that I got re-orientated and that was because, actually, in my field journal you can see that there was a level of tension and expectation about me going back in there, and that was about my being in a very different role . . . I was aware that even though I'd talked to people about the fact that I was coming back as a researcher, for most people, as soon as they saw me, I was Anne the social worker not Anne the researcher. So it gave me a chance to re-orientate myself and other people to that new role. It also gave me a chance to see clearly what I suspected, that there were some spaces in the Valley that already were shared public spaces, where in fact homeless people and mainstream community people did have a reasonable level of interaction, but that those spaces had changed in the four years that I hadn't been working in the Valley. It gave all sorts of people a chance to get used to me and that was really important . . . One of the things that happened all the time was that constantly people would come up to me and say, 'What are you doing? What's in the book? What are you writing down there?' A lot of them were homeless people I knew but a great number of them were just local people who felt that this was their space too and they wanted to know who I was, writing in this book, and what I was writing about . . .

Informal interviews in public spaces

Anne: Phase two was like the active engagement—I was in those public spaces I'd identified in the first phase and my purpose was to talk to anybody that used those spaces. 'What do you think about this place? What do you like about the Valley? Why do you come here? Is it interesting? Does it make you feel scared?' Anything that people wanted to tell me about the Valley, I wanted to hear . . . So in between encounters I'd be sitting down taking some notes and if I was just sitting around looking for some interesting people to have a talk to I'd be taking a note of what I was seeing. So it

	wasn't strictly observational though observation happened.
Yvonne:	So how did that phase differ in terms of its purpose from the first phase?
Anne:	The major difference was its focus . . . In the first phase, what was motivating me and the focus of my attention was the space itself. In the second phase, the focus was people . . .
Yvonne:	And what were the benefits of that second stage?
Anne:	I became much more confident. Probably because all of that initial stuff about being the observer had largely been resolved so I wasn't getting interrupted. People didn't come up and ask me what I was doing any more . . . It was also just another look at things before I started in-depth interviews with homeless people and the more I saw before I went into those interviews obviously the better the interviews were going to be.

Anne went back for a second stage of observation towards the end of the study, even though she had not initially planned to do so.

Anne:	After I did the in-depth interviews I thought I was finished until I went back and did the feedback, but there'd been some very interesting and quite significant things that had happened in the Valley while I was doing the in-depth interviews and I wanted to go back and capture what these were about.

Knowing when to stop

Yvonne:	When did you start to feel that you had enough data?
Anne:	Even before I got to the end of the in-depth interviews, there was a real commonality that was starting to surface . . . I was starting to hear the same sorts of things from, you know, police [who] were saying things about people who have been here in the community—they identified 'homeless people' as being local community as opposed to 'itinerants' who are outside people—but I started to hear the same sorts

of things from homeless people about how they perceived themselves. So even though I was getting it from a different point of view, the same sort of stuff was being replicated across different groups and across different homeless people. So it was all starting to converge. Also, I knew that there was still a feedback phase to come and if I'd missed anything major people would say at that stage, 'Hey wait a minute', so there was nothing lost that couldn't be got back. So I felt quite satisfied and somewhat relieved.

Timing, duration and recording

Anne: I couldn't do any more than about two hours at a time because I couldn't absorb it and I couldn't hold it in my memory if I went much over that. So I'd jot down what were basically memory prompts while I was in the field for that two hours. I'd then leave and if I was going straight home, I'd sit down at the computer and start to write up a set of notes based on the ones I'd taken in the field. If there was going to be a delay then I'd go somewhere private and fill the initial notes out, and then write them up as soon as I got home.

Yvonne: So for two hours observing, generally speaking, how long would that take you to write up your notes?

Anne: Anywhere from—if it had been a quiet day, there hadn't been a lot of people round, there hadn't been much happening—maybe two hours. But some days, writing up the field notes would take four hours. Sometimes, if there was more complicated stuff going on, or if anything I'd observed had had a big impact, there'd be another couple of hours of journal time because I also kept a separate journal to record my feelings and also to process, I guess, methodological decisions that I made as I went along. But part of the reason in the end that I kept observation periods to two hours was because I couldn't keep up with writing them up.

Yvonne: Did you vary the time of day that you observed?

84

Anne: Another useful thing I picked up in the first observational phase was that public spaces in Fortitude Valley
change and they can literally change in the movement
of a hand. If you were looking in the opposite direction you'd completely miss it. So at one minute a
space can be where this particular group is and this
is happening. Five minutes later—totally different
groups of people, totally different things happening. So
I was clear from pretty early on that I had to consider
the 24-hour clock and that I had to be aware of what
went on all through that clock. So that's what I did. I
think in the end the night stuff was under-represented.
There was a total of somewhere between 120 and 150
hours and probably only about a third of those hours
were night-time hours. So it was definitely weighted
on the day-time side but I still spent enough time at
night observing to have a clear idea about what went
on and I could identify when the transition times
across the 24 hours were, when those changes
happened, what groups came in and out. So, I think
that was a solid enough picture to work from.

Keeping homeless people informed about the study

Anne used an innovative approach to keeping in contact with this
population, to let people know she wanted to conduct some in-
depth interviews, to advertise her feedback sessions and, generally,
to let anyone who was interested know that she was still around
and involved in the research. Here, she talks about how she let
people know that she wanted to do some interviews.

Anne: I put a flier out saying that I wanted to do interviews
with people and why . . . I kept the words to a
minimum and I put a graphic on it that after a while
every time somebody saw something with that graphic
on, they'd go, 'Oh this is a thing about Anne's
research.' So even people who couldn't read knew
that this was a bona fide communication about this
particular piece of research. The graphic was just one
of those standard ones you get in computer packages,

but it was a suitcase being opened up and out of the suitcase were springing all these high-rise buildings. So, it kind of captured my sense of what was happening for these people. This is your local area, this is your home, you open it up and now look what's springing up out of it. So, the graphic became a sort of signal all the way through. If there was any communication I wanted to make with people, that went on the top of it. And people who weren't literate then would say to people, 'Here's one of Anne's fliers, like what's happening, what's going on?', so people who couldn't read were able to be involved as well.

Cheryl Tilse—The long goodbye

Cheryl's study of the experiences of older people who had placed a partner in a nursing home used several methods. She first conducted in-depth interviews with nine men and nine women who had recently placed a partner in a nursing home or a dementia hostel. She began with in-depth interviews as her concern was very much with trying to understand the perspectives of the spouses. She then used the six units in which they had placed their partners as a focus for observation of how visitors were treated and provided for. She also conducted brief, semi-structured interviews with staff about how they viewed visitors, and did a content analysis of any documents that the nursing home had produced for or about families.

Here Cheryl talks about her use of observation as a data collection method. She has published two papers on her use of participant observation in this study (Tilse, 1997a; 1997b) and has also reported on the themes from her in-depth interviews with spouses (Tilse, 1994).

Choosing observation

Yvonne: How did you come to choose observation as one of your data collection methods?

Cheryl: It was partly a commitment to try to understand the complexity of the experience and my view that you couldn't understand how family visitors were provided for and treated without actually being in the setting . . . I also had a theoretical interest in the use of space to include and exclude people in health settings . . . I also wanted to watch interactions between staff and families, and between families and other families. I wanted to understand whether visiting was primarily individual and private or whether it was social and collective. You could only understand [that] by watching what visitors did and how they interacted and how staff interacted with them. So I guess it was based on an understanding that what people say they do is often different to what happens . . . In residential care policy at that time there was a big interest in families. And part of the outcome standards was about being open to visitors and welcoming visitors and home-like environments. So there was a whole lot of rhetoric about families and I guess that was the other reason I wanted to observe because I didn't want to pick up the rhetoric. If I just interviewed staff, I thought there was the risk of [obtaining] socially desirable responses.

Observation role

Yvonne: If you can imagine a continuum between the complete observer and the complete participant, where were you along that line? And did that change at all during the course of the observations?

Cheryl: I was always clear that I was an observer, not a partic- ipant, in the sense that I didn't have a relative in the unit. I was saying, 'I'm not a staff member of the unit and I'm not a resident of the unit so I really am an observer and what I've come here to do is observe one feature of life—the treatment of family visitors'. So I really wasn't part of the place or pretending to be part of the place. I set myself up as a researcher, carried a notebook and made notes very overtly. I wanted to be seen as a researcher, as ethically I felt I had to be. And I also felt it provided lots of opportunity for people to say, 'What are you doing?', and I'd tell them and say, 'Well, what's it like to be a visitor?' So I had a way in to talk to people that I wouldn't have been comfortable with if I was pretending to be a staff member. So at that level I was very clearly an observer—ethically and researchwise . . . For most of it I sat and observed and listened and watched. I was keen to observe from a distance as I wasn't actually interested in what people said to each other—more [in] how the space was used and how people got included or excluded. So I kept myself at quite a distance from most interactions. I guess occasionally I felt I was a participant in that I was there and somebody with dementia would come up and start talking to me and I would have to respond, especially if the staff were running a particular activity. I would then try and help the resident join in the activity. So you would find yourself engaged in that sort of thing. With visitors as well. Some of the visitors would come over and say, 'What are you doing? This is really interesting. Come and have a talk to us.' And I would engage through talking and being part of their visiting and meeting their family. So you did get engaged in that way but it was always very clear to me and I tried to make it very clear to staff that I was just observing visitors. I wasn't doing anything else. But I also had to say I was a participant in that I'm visiting and experiencing all of this—I can't find a place to sit and I've been here all day and the tea trolley just passed me by . . . So I was a participant at that level. So it's always more messy in practice than it is in theory.

Yvonne: You said that you were very overt about your observing—you had your notebook and you were in a sense on view—but also that you tended to sit away from direct interactions. Did people always know they were being watched?

Cheryl: Probably not. I asked staff to tell any visitors that I was on the unit and what I was there for and I left material. But people came in and were talking to staff members about an issue and then they were gone and I'm sure that they weren't aware that I was there. It was

88

interesting because I spent the whole—as much as
I could—almost the whole shift there. I was there for
a long time and I did become part of the furniture and
I noticed staff would suddenly say to me, 'Oh you're
still here?' . . . so I think they did lose track of the fact
that I was there, particularly in some of the units
where they were busy with bathing and showering
and I was just sitting in the dayroom and there were
other visitors in the dayroom; and the fact that I'm a
woman, and it was quite a feminine environment in
terms of residents, visitors and staff. I did come to slip
into the furniture or the shrubbery at times.

Timing of the observations

Yvonne: I'm interested in the timing and duration of your observations. You've said you observed on all three shifts?

Cheryl: What I did was try to sample the shifts when visitors
were most likely to come. So I'd stay three or four
hours. I think they were six-hour shifts . . . So I didn't
go at six in the morning when they were showering
and feeding people when they told me that no visitors
came. I came in the afternoons, sort of mid- to late
afternoon, and they used to say no visitors come after
seven and that was true. The time I slept over in the
nursing home there were no visitors. So it wasn't
the whole shift but it was what they told me was the
most likely time there'd be visitors on the unit because
I made it very clear to them I wasn't observing care. I
think that was important in terms of their trust, that
I was really interested in observing visitors and the unit
in relation to visitors . . .

Yvonne: In hindsight what would you say would be an
optimum period of observation?

Cheryl: It depends on what you're observing and the depth of
what you're trying to understand so it's really hard to
say. I think after more than three hours you must start
to lose material. I had a whole lot of things that I was
looking at so I'd draw the setting and then when
visitors came I'd often draw, this is visitor one, and I'd

watch where they went. They ended up there and then how long they stayed and who talked to them . . . Often I had different diagrams for different visitors because it got very complicated but it was that sort of level of observation that kept me engaged. I wasn't trying to look at how residents were being treated. It was quite focused on one particular thing.

Yvonne: There must have been so much going on. Were there times when you saw things that were interesting but had to say to yourself, 'Well, that's really interesting but it's not what I'm here to look at'? Were you able to focus yourself in that way?

Cheryl: Yes. It wasn't that intense, I guess, in most places. So occasionally a whole lot of visitors came at once . . . but it was the fact that I was only trying to observe simple things, like did they speak to the registered nurse. I had a whole list of things I was interested in. One was the use of space. One was entry and exits. How did they enter, who did they talk to . . . But most of the time it wasn't high intensity. It was over a fair spread of time. The work for the workers was very busy but in fact for the visitors it was quite a slower pace. People came and stayed a few hours so I could see. They sat there on the verandah for two hours and it wasn't something that you would miss.

Recording the observations

Yvonne: I'd like to ask you now about recording. You used diagrams and had some broad categories—how structured was that and were there other ways you recorded?

Cheryl: I wanted something that was obvious note-taking but not too obtrusive and clearly not tape recorders or anything like that. I used those little shorthand notebooks because on one side I'd put clear descriptions and the other side of the page I kept for analytical or interpretative notes or questions I had to follow-up— 'This appears to be happening; I should check this out'. So I kept my analysis and ongoing interpretation of questions separate from pure description. I had a notebook for each unit. So I'd just record at the start the date, the time I arrived, the unit I was on, the shift and then I would write down what I saw. But it was always important, because I had this thing about space, to draw diagrams of who was where so I could remember it when I was analysing what was happening—to remember how long people spent out on the verandah without a staff member speaking to them.

Comments

An important message from both these examples is that observation can tell us things that other methods of data collection can't. Observation enables us to see events and interactions as they unfold, not filtered through someone else's perception of what is happening. It is those perceptions, of course, that observation cannot tell us about, hence the common practice in qualitative research of combining observation and interviews.

The examples also highlight the central roles of the observer, as both a filter of what is recorded and a part of the research context. Only what the observer notices and decides is relevant is recorded, and the observer in turn has an impact on the observational environment. Assumptions and biases need to be stated; while what is observed will always be filtered through the observer's mindset, it is also possible to take steps to minimise bias and inaccuracy in observation. Being conceptually clear about what is being observed can assist rigour and consistency in observation, as can taking seriously the physical limits of one's capacity to observe and later record.

In the following chapter, we consider some ways in which data collection approaches may be modified to suit the needs of particular groups of research participants.

5

Tailoring data collection to suit the needs of research participants

The data collection processes we have talked about so far are applicable to qualitative research with any group. In this chapter, we consider how data collection processes may need to be modified to suit the needs of particular groups, using children and people with an intellectual disability as examples.* We are *not* saying that all children and all people with an intellectual disability require a different approach to data collection. These groups are far too diverse to suggest that one approach would fit all for a start, and in many cases research with these groups will be no different from that with any other group. Rather, our position is that some children (the less so the older they are) and some people with an intellectual disability (the less so the milder the difficulty) will require particular efforts to be made by the researcher to promote their full and active participation. Some of the material in this chapter will also be relevant to research with people suffering cognitive impairment as a result of conditions such as stroke, dementia or acquired brain injury. Knowledge of particular conditions and their cognitive effects on the individual is obviously important if the researcher is to make the adaptations necessary to achieve the best possible communication with the research participant.

* In this book, we mainly use the terms 'intellectual disability' and 'people with an intellectual disability' which are the preferred current Australian nomenclature. We acknowledge that other terms, such as 'learning disability', 'developmental disability' or 'learning difficulty', are used in other contexts.

We focus here particularly on practical aspects of engagement with research participants and data collection. Ethical issues, particularly in relation to obtaining informed consent, have been considered in Chapter 2.

Both children and people with an intellectual disability have, until relatively recently, remained 'voiceless' in the research literature. They have been overlooked as potential research participants, considered either too vulnerable to be troubled by researchers, or to be unreliable sources of information. It is not that children and people with an intellectual disability have been under-researched per se, but that they have had limited opportunities to speak on their own behalf—parents, teachers, carers and case records have all been prefered as sources of information about them.

Children's rights and disability rights movements have, in recent times, played an important role in highlighting, and attempting to redress, the absence of voices of children and people with an intellectual disability in research. An essential step is accepting that children and people with an intellectual disability do have important things to say on their own behalf, and that their perspectives are a valuable source of input into decisions regarding themselves as individuals and the development of services more generally.

This is only a first step. Another hurdle to the inclusion of children and people with an intellectual disability in research concerns the skills of the researchers working with these groups. Researchers have too often avoided including these groups as research participants, considering them too hard to get information from or unable to express a point of view, and instead asking others to speak on their behalf. Researchers may have feared intruding or doing the wrong thing, and held concerns that participation could be detrimental. In many cases, they may just not have known how to work directly with children or with people with an intellectual disability. Researchers' lack of skill in working with these groups can be addressed, either through the researcher acquiring the necessary skills or through working in a team with someone who already has these skills.

The remainder of this chapter focuses separately on the practicalities of working with children and with people with an intellectual disability in the research context.

Researching with children

There is increasing recognition of children's rights to be involved in decisions affecting them. Just how and to what extent this should happen is a subject of continuing debate. Perspectives on children's rights range from liberationist views which focus on children's similarities to adults, and thus argue for expanded rights for children, to a protectionist stance that takes account of children's differences from adults as well as what they have in common, and seeks to preserve the differences, in the best interests of children (Wilkinson, 1993; Brannen & O'Brien, 1995).

The United Nations Convention on the Rights of the Child (United Nations Centre for Human Rights, 1989) steers a middle course in that it 'embraces both the vulnerable, dependent child requiring special protection and also the child who is a potential adult, or is adult-like, and thus the rightful recipient of a range of civil, political, legal and social rights similar to those attaching to the status of adult (Carney, 1991)' (Wilkinson, 1993, p. 148).

Article 12.1 of the Convention is germane to practice in areas such as family law, child protection and education, and is also relevant to the research context:

> States Parties shall assure to the child who is capable of forming his or her own views the right to express those views freely in all matters affecting the child, the views of the child being given due weight in accordance with the age and maturity of the child.

In this section, we draw together some of the considerable practice wisdom that has developed in research with children, in particular on interviewing and conducting participant observation with children. In this discussion, we in no way view children, even those of similar ages, as homogenous groups about whom rigid generalisations can be made. Fixed age-related stages of children's cognitive development and their use and understanding of language are being increasingly challenged (Donaldson, 1978; Carey, 1985; Keil, 1989). Donaldson, for example, emphasises the situational context of children's cognitive and language capacity, suggesting that children are generally more likely to display competence when they are 'dealing with "real-life" meaningful situations in which they have purposes and intentions and in which they can recognise and respond to similar purposes and intentions in others' (1978, p. 121). Thus, both the behaviour of others and what is expected of them need to make sense to them.

The experiences of researchers who have worked with children are presented here as a guide to some approaches that may be useful, not as recipes for how to work with children. In the final analysis, the 'best' thing to do has to be worked out in the context of the individual relationships between the researcher and each child. There are, however, a couple of overriding principles in working with children, in any context. These are the importance of neither over-estimating nor under-estimating a child's capabilities, and the necessity to like children, to be comfortable with them, to be really interested in what they think and feel, and to be able to communicate this to them.

Interviewing children

In this section, we consider first the issue of deciding who to interview and in what order. This is important in studies where other family members are also being interviewed. We then consider some practical issues relating to the interview context itself.

Who to interview and in what order?

In research with children there will always be adults whose cooperation and trust, as well as formal consent, is crucial to the child's participation in the research. Very often, others who are significant in the child's life will also be interviewed. Researchers have taken a number of approaches to deciding the order in which interviews are conducted, or whether to interview children alone or with others. There is no right or wrong approach. All have pros and cons, and these are decisions that need to be made in the context of the research purpose and the setting in which it is being conducted.

In general, where parents and children are being interviewed, interviewing parents first gives them an opportunity to get to know the interviewer and also to develop a clear idea of what the interviews involve. In all cases, parents should be informed as to the nature of the children's interviews, and any techniques that will be used. It is also vital that they understand the importance of not influencing what the children say, both prior to the initial interview and before any subsequent interviews.

Interviewing the parents first may also alert the interviewer to any indicators that children may later be exposed to pressure by a parent to disclose what they said in an interview. This may be especially so in research on sensitive topics such as separation or divorce; at times a decision may have to be made as to whether or not to proceed with a child's interview.

In a study on contact after divorce in which both parents and at least one child were interviewed, Trinder, Beek and Connolly (2001) used separate interviewers for each member of the family. All the children's interviews were conducted by a social worker experienced in working with children and others on the team alternated between interviewing mothers and fathers. While this approach would not prevent a parent intent on asking children what they had said from doing so, it at least established a sense of the importance of each having their own say, separate from what others might have said.

Interviewing parents and children together may help deal with parents' concerns about what is being asked of children, but may pose other difficulties. Hood, Kelley and Mayall (1996; see also Mayall, 1999) found the presence of adults at times altered the behaviour of all concerned—the interviewer, the child and the parent. Very often the interviews ended up largely as exchanges between the adults, even though the child's perspective was the major focus of the research. Analysis of transcripts revealed interviewers deferring to and siding with parents' views, interviewers keeping firmly to their own research agenda rather than taking the time to follow the child's view, parents interrupting and speaking for children, children struggling to be heard among the adult voices, children deferring to adults' views, and children presenting a united front, with parents, in relation to any questioning about intergenerational issues within the family.

The interview

As with any interview situation, the context of an interview with a child will shape the interaction. Children need an emotionally supportive environment if they are to feel comfortable enough to participate in an interview. It is important to take the time to develop a friendly and informal relationship with the child, and to make the interview context as child-focused as possible. This can be achieved through using a venue, context and reporting media familiar to the child, and allowing the child as much control over the process as possible, such as choosing to participate, choosing the venue and activities, and stating when they want to stop.

In a study of children's perceptions of harm and risk, their own anxieties and their experiences of adult support and professional intervention, Butler and Williamson (1994) interviewed 190 children within and outside the protective care system. They aimed to allow children as much control as possible in the interview situation, through giving them the choice of being interviewed singly, in pairs or in small groups, and putting them in control of the tape recorder and the duration of the interview.

Tammivaara and Enright suggest getting away from a straight question-and-answer format as children will perceive this as an examination-like context and provide what they perceive to be the right kind of answers for this context. They also suggest letting children direct the interview process as far as possible. At times this will involve the adult letting go of their adult control and authority and 'playing dumb' in order to let the child set the adult right and really try to get the adult to understand what they mean: 'Once the ethnographer is established as a "dummy" in need of guidance (a lasting "one-down" status), the child informant will often provide explanations and information voluntarily and at almost any time in or out of the formal interview encounter' (Tammivaara & Enright, 1986, p. 231).

In a study of children's ideas about health, Backett and Alexander (1991) commenced their child interviews with discussion of drawings the children had done prior to the interview. They had sent four- to twelve-year-old children a drawing pad prior to the interview, asking them to 'Draw all the things you yourself do that make you healthy and keep you healthy'. Parents were given advice on how to encourage the child, without influencing their drawing. Beginning the interviews in this way enabled the children to talk about something they were already familiar with, set them at ease, and provided a focus for the interview content.

Another way to maximise children's comfort in the research setting is to combine data collection with another activity that is already familiar to the child. Tammivaara and Enright (1986) suggest using classroom settings such as 'show and tell'; asking teachers to include questions as part of everyday activities (such as classroom discussion on a particular topic); or to use familiar game routines within interviews (such as asking children to make up a story or draw a scene, or to play 'let's pretend'). Similarly, Backett and Alexander suggest, 'Keep the interviews open, flexible and structured around the daily experiences of the child' (1991, p. 35). Whatever choices are made about how to interview children, contextual issues should be discussed thoroughly and transparently in reports on the research. This includes anything about the way the research was conducted that could have affected the children's responses or performance, such as the timing of the interviews, the venue, the activities, what choices the children had, or who else was present.

Siegert (1986) raises some interesting issues in relation to the process of interviewing children and the nature and quality of data obtained. In discussing research on children's social competence, he argues that an interview between an adult and a child can legitimately tell us a lot about children's competences in adult–child interaction, in contexts defined by adults, but it is questionable whether that can be generalised to other contexts, for example with peers. Siegert suggests that a combination of participant observation and group discussions among children would be more appropriate ways to gather data about peer interactions.

In research on children's perspectives, it is important to take the lead from the child as to what they find interesting enough to talk about (Beresford, 1997). This avoids making assumptions about what the researcher thinks might be most interesting and relevant to them or holding too firmly on to one's own topic list of what seems to be important. Beresford also suggests taking the time to establish the words and phrases used by the child at the beginning of the interview and using the child's language.

In the context of child abuse investigations, Steward, Bussey, Goodman and Saywitz suggest that in order to maximise children's communication:

> The interviewer should listen to the child's narrative report, not only for the content, but also for the child's spontaneous use of language. The interviewer should then match his/her own sentence length and complexity to the child's in order to maximize the communication. Interviewers can assume that the younger the child, the shorter the sentences the child will comprehend, the fewer verb-noun units per utterance, the fewer syllables per word and the more they will depend on familiar contextual cues to glean meaning (Steward et al., 1993, pp. 32–3).

Making use of pictures, books and other props also gives children something to do, taking the pressure off the verbal interaction. Tammivaara and Enright say: 'Young children generally find doing something with something and talking about that something to be easier, more comfortable, and more interesting than only talking about something that isn't physically present (i.e. an event, a routine, an idea)' (1986, p. 232).

Group discussions and focus groups

Group discussions or focus groups can be used as a variation on individual interviews. The group context may well be more familiar and less intimidating than the individual interview, and can be a useful way of encouraging more reticent children to offer information they might not provide in an individual interview (Mates & Allison, 1992; Hoppe et al., 1995; Beresford, 1997). Topics with the potential to cause discomfort or embarrassment for any child in the group should, however, be reserved for individual interviews or pencil and paper exercises.

Hoppe et al. (1995) used focus groups with primary school age children to develop measures for a study about children's knowledge and understanding of HIV and AIDS. The focus groups assisted them to understand children's level of knowledge, and the language they used to discuss these and related topics. They recommend groups of five, as it was difficult to get lively discussion going with smaller groups, and with six or more it became difficult to hold the attention of the group and to draw out quieter children. They also recommend homogeneity of age and gender, use of moderators experienced in working with children, and sessions of one hour or less. They found it useful to move from less sensitive to more sensitive topics and to avoid abstract questions, instead asking concrete questions that led children to talk about their own experience. They also suggest making the setting as informal and unschool-like as possible, and spending some time 'warming up' and getting to know the children.

Participant observation with children

Fine and Sandstrom (1988) provide an excellent introduction to participant observation with children of various ages; we draw on their work in the following discussion.

The role the adult observer takes vis-à-vis the child will be a powerful shaper of the research, and of what children will allow the observer to see and/or to participate in. While some suggest that the adult observer can divest themselves of their 'adultness' and so interact with children as an equal (Goode, 1986), or in a least-adult way (Mandell, 1988), Fine and Sandstrom recommend the researcher take the middle ground, in the role of an adult friend:

> The final major type of participant observation role, and the one emphasised in this book, is to become a friend to one's subjects and interact with them in the most trusted way possible—without having any explicit authority role. As indicated above, in our view, this will always be an ideal type because of the demographic and power differences involved . . . We believe there is a methodological value in maintaining the differences between sociologists and children—a feature of interaction that permits the researcher to behave in certain 'nonkid' ways—such as asking 'ignorant' questions (Fine & Sandstrom, 1988, p. 17).

In a participant observation study of pre-schoolers' peer behaviour, Corsaro (1985) chose a 'reactive' approach to engaging with the children. He was present and available in the children's activity areas, but waited for them to make the first moves. After some initial tentative advances from a couple of children, they gradually seemed to accept his presence and involvement in their activities. While clearly not 'one of them', the children also did not regard him as a formal authority figure, responding to his occasional attempts to control their behaviour with 'You're not a teacher' or 'You can't tell us what to do' (1985, p. 31).

Even so, any adult will inevitably be seen to some extent as an authority figure, and issues of children's reactivity to an adult presence need to be taken into account (Fine & Sandstrom, 1988). It is important that the adult participant–observer has some reason for being there that is understood and accepted by the children, as a first step to developing a relationship with them. The researcher's presence and where they fit in needs to make sense to the children. Establishing rapport with adult authorities or caregivers is also essential, especially where the researcher holds no formal authority in relation to the children.

Fine and Sandstrom suggest that observation is possible with children from age three, when 'the child begins to belong to a group that is meaningful to him or her, and, as a consequence, group relations can be studied' (1988, p. 36). While consent for children to participate in research must be obtained from parents, they recommend that even young children be given as much information as possible about the research and the role of the researcher: 'Perhaps the children should be told that there will be an adult who will watch and play with them to learn what they like and what they do. This simple explanation might be sufficient to provide a measure of informed consent consistent with the informants' understanding' (1988, p. 46).

Older children are in a much better position to vote with their feet—both in terms of whether they agree to be part of the research and, as it proceeds, to control the researcher's access to their activity, even where adults have already given consent to the researcher's presence. Provided the researcher does not also hold a formal authority role in relation to them, older children can decide whether or not to trust this person and have a measure of control over what aspects of their worlds they will allow the researcher to participate in and/or to observe.

> The preadolescents had the authority to decide when I could be present, in ways in which the preschoolers would never conceive. This power means that preadolescents will have a fair degree of authority to shape the role of the researcher, and the researcher who wishes to gain rapport with informants must recognize this (Fine & Sandstrom, 1988, p. 50).

While older children may find ways to control what the researcher does and doesn't observe, certainly what they do and do not participate in, participant observation, by its very nature, is structured by the researcher—with decisions about where to observe, what issues to focus on, what to look for, and so on resting with the researchers. Mayall (1999) suggests ongoing consultation with children as the research progresses and using their input on interim findings in the development of later stages of the research. This at least gives the children being researched some opportunity to comment on what the researcher has made of their activity and, if necessary, to clarify the meaning of what has been observed.

Involving children in the research process

While examples of children forming an active part of the research team are relatively rare, there is increasing recognition of the importance of understanding more about children's experiences if we are to develop educational and social programs and services that adequately meet their needs.

One example of children being actively involved as researchers is an edited book of the teaching and learning approach of Cleves School in London (Alderson, 1999). The school had a reputation for being a model for inclusive education and independent and group learning, and Alderson was funded to work with the staff and children on writing a book about their school. A team of Year 6 students participated actively in the writing committee. The committee decided what topics would be included in the book and conducted interviews throughout the school of people's experiences—as students, teachers and parents.

Hill, Laybourn and Borland's (1996) study of children's perceptions of their emotional needs and well-being was conducted in order to develop health education materials aimed at helping adults to be more responsive and supportive towards children, and subsequently formed the basis for an information leaflet for parents (Health Education Board for Scotland 1997, cited in Borland, et al., 1998). The researchers conducted focus groups and interviews with children aged five to twelve. A similar approach was used for both, with a variety of structured activities, both verbal and non-verbal, but including various points at which 'children were asked to specify or make choices about the issues to be discussed' (Hill et al., 1996, p. 133). The researchers clearly saw this as a compromise position, maximising children's input into the research, but having to work within time and resource constraints.

Even where children are not actually engaged in the research process, it is important, wherever possible, to provide feedback to the children after data analysis as a check against possible misinterpretation of the information they provided (Beresford, 1997).

Researching with people with an intellectual disability

Working with people with an intellectual disability presents a real challenge for qualitative researchers as this, more than any other, is a talking research. Qualitative researchers like to really understand what various life experiences and events mean to people and thus we tend to prize highly articulate and reflective research participants. Even when observation represents a significant part of data collection, we most often also want to talk with people, to check out what we have observed and to find out what the activity we have observed means to those involved. Undertaking qualitative research with people with an intellectual disability thus requires at least three things. First, that we value the experiences of those who are not as articulate or verbal as we are; second, that we accept their experience of themselves and their world as valid—and not as either inferior or a threat to our own way of being in the world; and finally, that we find ways to elicit their experience, for their voices to be heard. This section offers some suggestions for ways of communicating verbally with people with an intellectual disability, in the research context. We acknowledge that this field is still evolving and that there is developing knowledge and experience with research participants who have non-verbal means of communication.

Understanding participants and their context

In any research with people with an intellectual disability, Biklen and Moseley (1988) recommend an initial period of observation prior to interviewing. This will assist the researcher's understanding of the research participants and their situation, provide a safeguard against making incorrect assumptions about the level of communication that is or is not possible and may also assist participants to become familiar with the researcher's presence. Where possible, observation should take place in a variety of settings, both formal and informal. Official records and accounts from significant others of the person's life history and preferences can also be used as supplementary sources of information (Biklen & Moseley, 1988).

Interviewing

Interviews are best conducted in a familiar environment, preferably of the participant's choosing and at a pace suitable to them. A series of brief meetings may be more effective than relying on one formal interview (Booth & Booth, 1994a, 1994b; Biklen & Moseley, 1988). In some situations, inclusion of a person well known to the informant may be a useful way to handle language difficulties and communication problems, though they should always be well briefed about the purpose of the research and the importance of obtaining the respondent's own perspective. Some people will be better at this than others. Some will filter out important parts of the story, others embellish it with their own perspectives; their presence may also constrain what the respondent reports (Biklen & Moseley, 1988). Booth and Booth (1994b) found joint interviews with significant others were sometimes useful in opening up discussion but also carried the risk that the respondent's voice was excluded if a more articulate significant other took over.

A compromise approach is to have participants interviewed by someone they know who is, at the same time, independent of the research topic. Minkes, Robinson and Weston (1994), for example, used teachers to interview children with an intellectual disability about their experiences of residential respite care. The teachers already had rapport with the children, thus assisting them to relax in the interview situation, and were also able to interpret non-verbal responses.

In summary, getting to know the people you are working with and taking the lead from others who know them well and communicate effectively with them are invaluable principles in research with people with an intellectual disability.

We include here some specific approaches that researchers have found useful in interviewing people with an intellectual disability. These are by no means prescriptive, and in no way substitute for taking the time to get to know the people involved and their capabilities.

- Avoid comparison questions (for example, How are supervisors different from counsellors?); instead, ask about people, things and activities separately (Biklen & Moseley, 1988).
- Open-ended questions may elicit only one- or two-word answers. It is generally more effective to ask a series of specific questions separately, and so build up an incremental picture of what the informant thinks (Biklen & Moseley, 1988; Booth & Booth, 1994a, 1994b).
- The use of visual cues such as pictures and photographs can assist in eliciting information from children and adults with an intellectual disability (Minkes, Robinson & Weston, 1994) and are particularly useful in facilitating responses to open-ended questions (Booth & Booth, 1994a, 1994b).

Booth and Booth (1994a) also provide helpful suggestions for finding out about the time and frequency of events. In summary, they suggest:

- Settle for approximate times where these will suffice, for example, whether the duration of a relationship has been weeks or years.
- Wherever possible, find another marker, for example, whether something had happened before or after another whose date was known.
- Use their children as a chronometer—gauging other events in terms of how old the children were at the time.

Being flexible in data collection

If data collection is to be tailored to the needs and capacity of each participant, then flexibility of approach is inevitable. Here, qualitative methods are particularly appropriate. Not only is there less emphasis on standard questions and administration procedures than in quantitative research, but flexibility of approach and responsiveness to the context are very much part of good practice.

In a study of young people's experiences of special education, Wade and Moore used a structured questionnaire and open-ended sentence completions. Some students were able to complete the exercises on their own while others required assistance from teachers to read out statements and scribe responses. The researchers traded off potential 'contamination' of the data against enabling as many students as possible to express their views.

> We were aware that, in these cases, the guaranteed anonymity of a privately written response was removed, and students' responses might be modified to take account of the scriber as audience. The alternative was to exclude a substantial number of children whose disabilities precluded their making written responses but who were just as capable of expressing their views in other ways (orally or by signing, for example) (Wade & Moore, 1993, p. 21).

In their study of children's experiences of residential respite care, Minkes, Robinson and Weston (1994) used an interview/discussion format that could be used with all children, whether they communicated by speech or other means. The same questions were asked of all children, but for those who did not communicate easily by speech, several visual cues were used. These included photographs of the residential homes, staff members and other children, pictures of everyday objects and small books that could be used by the children and interviewers to develop a pictorial record of their experiences at the home (the children who did this were able to keep their book). Again, teachers used their existing knowledge of the children to devise imaginative ways of using the available cues.

Involving people with an intellectual disability in research

Linda Ward (1997) provides practical guidelines for involving disabled children and young people at every stage of research, from project development through to dissemination. Elsewhere, Ward and Simons (1998) describe several ways in which people with an intellectual disability have been able to participate in research processes, including: helping to shape the research agenda, through lobbying for research to be conducted on issues of importance to people with an intellectual disability; advising and assisting research projects; doing research themselves; and being involved in research dissemination.

Dissemination of research to people with an intellectual disability requires serious consideration of the form in which research results are presented. Researchers at the University of Bristol (Bashford, Townsley & Williams, 1995) have developed 'parallel texts' of research reports as a means of making research accessible to people with an intellectual disability. They include both the formal and complete report and a simplified version, not as a separate document, but in parallel form within the report, on facing sheets. They argue that providing access to both the original and the simplified versions helps to break down pervasive 'them' and 'us' attitudes and also avoids making judgements about the skill levels of those accessing the report. Any user of the research may read the simple or complete version or move between the two, according to their own levels of skill and interest in the report.

Stories from the field

In the following inside stories, Caroline Thomas talks about her research with adopted children, and Tim and Wendy Booth talk about their work with parents who have learning difficulties. These inside stories illustrate the ways in which some of the principles and techniques we have discussed in this chapter can be put into practice.

Caroline Thomas—Adopted children speaking

Caroline worked with a research team in Wales to find out about older children's experiences of the adoption process. The study focused on children who were adopted at the age of five or later and who had previously been looked after by the local authority. The study report, authored by Caroline Thomas and Verna Beckford, with Nigel Lowe and Mervyn Murch, is published as *Adopted Children Speaking* by the British Agencies for Adoption and Fostering (1999).

The study was one of a set of studies funded by the UK Department of Health specifically to contribute to an adoption law review in the early 1990s. Initially, research was commissioned in relation to adoptive parents, adoption agencies and post-adoptive services for older adopted children. This particular study was commissioned about two years into the larger series of studies, due to concern from the advisory group that children's perspectives were not being included.

Forty-one children were interviewed for the study. They were aged between eight and fifteen at the time of the interview, with 83 per cent aged between eight and twelve. All the interviews were conducted in the children's homes. Most of the children were interviewed alone, in private, but there were also three interviews with pairs of siblings, and six interviews where a parent was either present or within earshot. The interviews commenced with a warm-up period during which the interviewer obtained permission to tape, explained confidentiality, encouraged the children to nominate and rehearse a process by which they would indicate they wanted not to answer a particular question or to stop the interview and asked the children to sign a simple consent form. The children were then asked to create an 'eco map' of the families, friends and professionals involved in their lives. The third stage of the interview explored the children's experiences of the adoptive process and the help they had received during that process. In the end phase, children were offered certificates for taking part in the study and a personalised thankyou was sent later.

Caroline and her colleagues have reported the following insights from their research:

> From our direct experience of communicating with older adopted children during the interviews, and the views the children themselves

expressed about their understanding of adoption, life story work and contact issues, we learnt that it is particularly important for adults to:

- Express themselves simply and clearly and use concepts which are familiar to the children.
- Match their explanations of new ideas to the children's age and levels of understanding.
- Be aware of the possible impact of emotional distress on children's understanding.
- Elicit children's fears and offer reassurances.
- Allow children plenty of opportunities for asking questions.
- Ask children for feedback to see if information and explanations have been remembered and understood.
- Repeat, simplify, expand, or build on explanations if appropriate.
- Use communication tools such as games, prompt cards, books, videos and so on (Thomas et al., 1999, pp. 131–2).

Here, we talk with Caroline about choosing to conduct in-depth interviews with the children, the process of recruiting and engaging with the children, and the interviews.

Choosing a qualitative research approach

Caroline: We were sure that we needed a predominantly qualitative approach given that as far as we were aware adopted children's views about support hadn't been explored before. There wasn't anything to build on. It was exploratory. So we felt that that was the best approach given that situation.

We were encouraged to consider including some sort of assessment of the children's well-being . . . but Verna and I felt uncomfortable about that, partly because we didn't have the training to use psychometric tests. At that time, we didn't have the training to administer them, and didn't have the training to interpret them. While we would have been very happy to involve and engage other people in helping us, we thought we would be losing some control of the study by doing that and also we wondered what we would be learning. We would have learned that these were children who had emotional and behavioural difficulties and whose well-being wasn't too high up on the scale. We already knew that. What we didn't know was what they thought about what they had been through and what they remembered about it. That was what we really wanted to get at and focus upon.

Dorothy: So you really had to justify to others the choice of in-depth interviewing as the method?

Caroline: Yes. What also concerned us was . . . we had a certain budget which only allowed us to visit the children once and we were anxious about the amount of interview time [involved] in using a battery of tests. Had we included tests, the interviews would have been a wholly different experience for the children and I think that that has definitely been borne out by other work I've done subsequently that has involved psychometric testing.

. I think we have to be extremely careful about what we put children through in the interview process. It's not just about the level of intrusion—it's about the length of time that interviews can take and the need to relate that to children's capacity to concentrate and stay with what they're talking about . . . On average, we were with the children speaking about their experiences of adoption for about an hour and a half, and that seemed quite long enough.

Recruiting and engaging the children

Dorothy: Can you say a little bit about the process of the research? Thinking of moving through the recruitment and engagement and finally the interviewing, how you found yourself adapting this because the research participants were children—can you say a little bit about your own thinking and how that unfolded?

Caroline: In the recruitment process what was absolutely key to Verna and to me was that it was the children we needed, but to get to them we had to get past their gatekeepers—their adoptive parents. We had to convince them of the worth of all that we were doing. But we also wanted to be sure that the children wanted to speak to us at the outset. It was absolutely crucial to us that we didn't pressure them and that we were giving them as much information as possible about us and the study. We wanted them to be clear about what we were expecting from them. The challenge there was to try to communicate that to them in one opportunity. But we also had to produce material that was going to appeal and make sense to a huge range of different children . . . That was the big challenge there. And, for instance, we thought about whether we needed to produce different materials for different ages, whether we needed different materials for boys and girls, and whether we needed to try to make them culturally sensitive. We did go through all those options, but finally came up with something that we were confident in, once we tested it out with other children who were about the same age and who were imagining themselves into the situation of the children who would be receiving the materials. They gave us the reassurance we needed that the materials we'd produced would be acceptable.

The interviews

Dorothy: You've written about adapting the interviewing [for each child], individualising the interviewing really to be able to engage and reach this child, rather than doing it in a standardised way. Is there anything that you would add to that?

Caroline: Possibly the book doesn't convey the differences in those individual interviews. I mean, from speaking to a 13- or 14-year-old girl who was extremely comfortable just talking to me and very relaxed and articulate—we could have gone on talking for much longer than two hours—to a little boy who was literally 'all over the place', physically and mentally. With him at one point I ended up playing *Bagatelle* in the middle of the interview. Then we went out into the garden and walked around the garden and played football for a little while before coming back and doing a little bit more of the interview. It was sometimes important to let go of the ambition of covering all that I wanted to cover, and to try to find just a little bit of the adoption process that the child could talk about.

Dorothy: What was most challenging about the interviewing itself?

Caroline: Possibly sometimes feeling as though I was moving into territory that I didn't want to explore and having to put the stoppers on—putting boundaries up to discourage disclosure about certain experiences that really we weren't interested in. That was quite challenging . . . On one or two occasions I had to respond to the children's distress about what they were talking about and wondered whether I had done that well enough. I wondered how the child felt after the interview was over and whether the adoptive parents would be able to pick up on any issues that were left over. So that was challenging. And I think that though I say that the need to be adaptive made the interviews interesting, it made some of the interviews extremely challenging. Sometimes it was hard just trying to follow the child, trying to get something from the interview for the study but at the same time not exploiting the child . . .

Dorothy: It's interesting that your concerns are not really about the research as a researcher but your concerns were fundamentally about the children as children—was that the hardest part, the most challenging area of the research?

Caroline: I think so, but it helped that after just a few interviews I was confident that the children's material was going to be rich enough for us to say some interesting things . . . so I was able to put aside people's concerns that we wouldn't be able to get something useful from the children.

Tim and Wendy Booth—Parenting under pressure

Tim and Wendy Booth's biographical study of the parenting experiences of people with learning difficulties was funded for two years by the Nuffield Foundation and is published as *Parenting*

Under Pressure: Mothers and Fathers with Learning Difficulties (1994a). Tim and Wendy have also reported on their use of in-depth interviewing with parents with learning difficulties (Booth & Booth, 1994b), on writing up narrative reports of inarticulate research participants (Booth & Booth, 1996) and on maintaining ongoing relationships with research participants (Booth, 1998). They have subsequently conducted a study of children of people with learning difficulties, published as *Growing Up with Parents who have Learning Difficulties* (Booth & Booth, 1998).

The study of parents was conducted in two stages. The first involved unstructured interviews with 33 parents, of whom 25 had learning difficulties, including five couples where both parents had learning difficulties, focusing specifically on experiences of parenthood. Six couples and one single parent then participated in the second stage, which involved the compilation of in-depth accounts of their ongoing situation as parents over the course of a year. The number of interviews in the first stage ranged from one to six, and in the second stage from nine to twenty. Both stages also involved numerous informal contacts such as brief social calls, phone calls and trips and outings with parents. In each family, at least one parent had at some stage received services especially intended for people with learning difficulties.

In their interview for this book, Tim and Wendy expanded on some of the points they have written about elsewhere. While we mostly rely on the interview material, we have also included some references to their published work.

Realising the need for a different approach

> *Wendy:* I always remember the very first interview where I went in with the idea of how I had been trained to do interviews. I would go in with an idea of the sort of questions I wanted to ask. We didn't have any formal questions. We just had an aide-mémoire. And I drew up outside the house and the door opened and the mother came out and greeted me and I went in and she was having a party. It was her birthday and the house was full of people and it was a case of just getting to know her in that situation really. And it was a really good introduction of how it was going to be

really because I wasn't able to record, write notes or anything, so I just had to remember what she was telling me. I learnt so much that day about that family. Her husband was there and her two children and all her friends . . . It was I guess a way of realising that I may as well forget all those ways I'd learnt, that this was going to be very different and I'm going to have to have new ways of talking to people.

Tim: It's a real challenge of methods here. How do you access people's stories? If you work from the textbook you get nowhere. They won't talk. They clam up. They'll parrot opinions, merely provide you with what they think you want to hear. Textbook methods won't work with this group of people so you have to be innovative and devise methods that will unlock the door. So that means a lot of experimentation, it means a lot of failure, until you hit the right button—and it's quite likely to be a different button with different people as well.

Taking the time to develop relationships

Tim and Wendy were very aware of the potential for exploiting people with an intellectual disability by offering a much-needed 'friendship' in order to get them to participate in the research.

Tim: These people have been subjected to endless assessments and measures that [very often] in the end have put them down in some way—they get referred to another school or they get debarred from going somewhere or they are referred somewhere they don't want to go . . . So you have to overcome that reticence before you can get people to talk and in doing that as well obligations come and it's important to recognise that. One doesn't want to end up in a situation where you're tricking people into talking by pretending you're a friend when all you're doing is using the guise of friendship to get information that serves your purpose. So the obligation from this method is recognition that there are reciprocal duties and responsibilities

113

here and that if as a friend people are giving you information, you have to take on the duties of friendship in return and honour those . . . So that means that at the end of the interview you can't just close the door and say goodbye and leave. If that's what people want, fair enough, but if people are expecting more of you than that, then the obligations, the kind of contract that you have established implicitly with them—you've got to honour those other ambitions . . . [To Wendy] In all of these studies, you've come out of them with some people who have wanted to stay in contact, so over the years, you've come out with a lot of friends who still get in touch, share problems, who sometimes just ring for a chat . . . I think in most other studies researchers would protect themselves against that sort of commitment by drawing clear boundaries around their role and saying this is what I am, this is what I'm doing, this is where it ends, but in truth, it's simply not possible to do that with this particular group of people because in order to grow that trust in which they feel free to talk honestly from the heart, you have to enter into a kind of relationship that goes beyond the straight researcher relationship . . .

I suppose that nowadays people describe things as participatory methods, and we have never particularly embraced that notion, but it is not an inaccurate description of what we did. Partly of course this wasn't us as researchers deciding to do it this way, it was dictated by the people that we were working with and by the way in which they conducted their own lives. The fact of the matter is that you would have rung up beforehand, you would have arranged an appointment for an interview, you would get there just as they were leaving the house, and you would say, 'Oh hi Jacqueline or John, I'm here', and they would say, 'Oh I had forgotten you were coming, I am just going to the shops', and so the only thing you could do is to quickly adapt and say, 'Is it all right if I come with you?'; 'Yes sure no problem' . . . So you would use that opportunity, the walk to the shops, the drive to the club that they were going to, go around the supermarket with them, and in the course of doing that, you are chatting and you would do what you intended to do in something as researchers we call an interview. You would do it on the hoof.

Approaches to interviewing

Tim and Wendy found that the parents in their study rarely took direction of the interviews themselves. They have said elsewhere:

> Generally speaking, our informants were more inclined to answer questions with a single word, a short phrase or the odd sentence . . . Although varying in their language skills, our informants' conversation tended to display some or all of the following characteristics: an instrumental rather than an expressive vocabulary; a present orientation; a concrete rather than an abstract frame of reference; a literal rather than a figurative mode of expression; a focus on people and things rather than feelings and emotions; and a responsive rather than a proactive style (Booth & Booth, 1994b, p. 421).

Given this, it seemed that developing trust was only part of the story. We were also interested to talk to Tim and Wendy about specific approaches they had used to elicit information from the parents.

Tim: We're back to the difference between textbook methods and methods in the real world. I mean, the textbooks will tell you not to ask leading questions, but if you don't ask leading questions with this group, you won't get any answers. What you need to know is enough about the person you're talking with to be able to judge the veracity of their replies. Let me give an example. Danny Avebury had no words [see Booth & Booth, 1996]. He replied to every question with one word, two words at most. His longest sentence in four and a half hours of interviewing was, 'Two rabbits and a ferret.' Otherwise he replied in monosyllables to whatever questions he was asked. But he couldn't lie. He always told the truth. He wasn't able to dissemble. So if you asked a leading question and he said yes or

115

no, you could be sure that his reply was an honest one, so you could build up a story, build up a picture of his life by either ruling things out, by getting him to say no to leading questions or by getting him to assent to one . . .

Yvonne: Thinking more about communication, one of the things that you talk about in your book is the importance of not patronising people with learning difficulties by pitching a discussion at too low a level. How do you work that out in any given interview situation?

Wendy: I suppose it is something that I do automatically now, so I am trying to remember what it was like to begin with. I think I have always gone in and talked to people as I would anybody else, and then gradually adjust the way I am talking, if I think they are not understanding me, to keep putting things in a different way and hoping that—not with everybody, sometimes you can still be misunderstood—even if you are asking in a very simple fashion . . . It is difficult to actually explain how you do that, but it's being able to pick up on key words that people use in their sentences. Somebody might only use sentences with four or five words in it, but you know that they are all very key words that they have picked— they don't have the grammar, but they can make their feelings known by those few words, so it doesn't really matter. If that is the conversation I am getting back, I could still talk to people in the way I would talk, and they could understand me, or I feel they can understand me, because of the way they are responding.

Yvonne: So the response is congruent with the question . . . Is there anything else on communication—on the practicalities of interviewing?

Tim: Use of photographs as props for interviews is very useful, particularly when you are in that first session, where you are just trying to get some idea of the family, of where people have come from, their background and history and that sort of thing, and asking people to show you their albums. You can work through family photographs, where they have them, as a very useful prop and I guess the other important thing here too is maintaining a concrete frame of reference in terms of the questions and how you progress the interview—not dealing with abstract notions. Being wary about things like time and people's ability to be able to place events in chronological sequence, but maintaining that focus, that concrete focus upon events that happened, what is, behaviour, specific examples—that is so important with this group of people.

Wendy: I think that is where it is important that you do know something about them, that you have taken the time to get to know them, because I know one mother who I would say does have very limited skills in communicating and if she says to me one word, like she would say the name of her newest grand-daughter, I know that she wants to talk about her and I can ask her a question, and she will come back, and it will only be very short sentences, but this is how we can communicate about it. As I have said before, just one or two really key words, and because you know them, you know what it is about, and then you can start having a conversation.

Comments

While these examples reflect very different research studies, both illustrate the importance of an individualised approach to working with research participants—taking the time to get to know and engage with research participants on their own terms. There is little point in relying on conventional notions of what happens in an interview if participants have neither previous experience of such a context nor a view of what an interview 'should' be like. Both research teams exercised considerable flexibility in their approach in order to elicit information about participants' experiences—whether abandoning an interview to play a game with a restless child or going shopping with a mother with a learning difficulty—and so were able to obtain a depth of understanding that would have been unlikely had they relied on a more conventional format.

Both studies also illustrate the importance of sensitivity to ethics and boundary issues. Caroline Thomas was careful not to take advantage of the children's ready trust, at times containing them from disclosure beyond her specific research brief, and Tim and Wendy Booth's ongoing involvement with research participants arose from their commitment to honouring reciprocal obligations to participants.

Along with increased expertise and willingness on the part of researchers to engage with children and people with an intellectual disability as research participants, there is also increasing recognition of the contribution these groups have to make as researchers, either in their own right or in partnership with research teams. We expect in the coming years to see many more instances of children and people with an intellectual disability taking a role in every stage of research that concerns them.

6

Mixing methods

'Mixed methods' is, in social science research, a shorthand way of saying that a study has combined qualitative and quantitative methods of data analysis. In this chapter we discuss studies that combine these methods in four common ways.

Mixing methods has been the subject of considerable debate in the social sciences and has variously been regarded as anathema, as the outcome of everyday pragmatic research decisions, or as appropriate in some situations but needing to be carefully justified. Greene, Caracelli and Graham (1989) identify three positions: the purists, the pragmatists and those taking a middle-ground, situationalist approach. At the one extreme are the purists, those who regard qualitative and quantitative methods as representing competing and incompatible paradigms, and for whom mixing is not tenable (Rist, 1977; Guba 1985; Smith & Heshusius, 1986; Guba & Lincoln, 1989). Guba (1985) says, 'We *are* dealing with an either-or proposition, in which one must pledge allegiance to one paradigm or the other; there is no compromise' (1985, p. 80).

The situationalists adhere to the notion of separate paradigms but value the increased understanding that can be obtained from examining aspects of social life from different perspectives (Filstead, 1979; Kidder & Fine, 1987; Oakley, 1999). Kidder and Fine say, 'We share the call for "synthesis", but at the same time, we want to preserve the significant differences between the two cultures. Instead of homogenizing research methods and cultures, we would like to see researchers become bicultural' (1987, p. 57). Similarly,

Filstead is adamant, on the one hand, that qualitative and quantitative methods 'represent fundamentally different epistemological frameworks for conceptualizing the nature of knowing, social reality, and procedures for comprehending these phenomena' (1979, p. 45), but he also argues for the inclusion of quantitative and qualitative methods to address different aspects of an evaluation, accepting that each may contribute to the strengthening of an evaluation design.

The pragmatists (e.g. Walker, 1985; Bryman, 1988, 1992; Miles & Huberman, 1994) tend to link choice of method directly to the research purpose and the questions being asked. As Walker says, 'Certain questions simply cannot be answered by quantitative methods, while others cannot be answered by qualitative ones' (1985, p. 16).

From a pragmatic stance, Bryman suggests that the epistemological differences between qualitative and quantitative research have become exaggerated. While he concedes that 'much of the exposition of the epistemological debts of qualitative research helped to afford it some credibility', he argues that in practice 'a great many decisions about whether and when to use qualitative methods seem to have little, if any, recourse to these broader intellectual issues' (1988, p. 108). The 'to mix or not to mix' debate has in fact abated somewhat in recent years, with the emergence of a more pluralistic approach in which methods are chosen on the basis of their suitability to address specific research needs.

It is perhaps not surprising that evaluation researchers have been prominent in debates and developments in mixed methods (Cook & Reichardt, 1979; Kidder & Fine, 1987; Mark & Shotland, 1987; Greene, Caracelli and Graham, 1989)—those commissioning evaluations are more likely to be concerned with getting answers to all the questions that interest them than with the ideological purity of how those answers are obtained.

Many research projects have a range of purposes incorporating several research questions. These questions may be primarily quantitative, primarily qualitative, or include both qualitative and quantitative elements. Questions that are either openly or implicitly about quantity, about how much or how many, or measuring one thing against another, are going to require quantitative analysis. Questions about meanings require qualitative analysis. We take the view that any combination or sequence of methods or approaches can be used, provided it can be justified by the research purpose and the different components are adequately articulated and integrated. This includes being clear about what each approach brings to the study, and their limitations.

There are many reasons why mixed methods may be appropriate. Greene, Caracelli and Graham (1989) reviewed 57 evaluation studies that used mixed methods and identified five main purposes for combining methods: triangulation; complementarity; development; initiation; and expansion.

• Triangulation seeks convergence, corroboration and correspondence of results from the different methods.
• Complementarity seeks elaboration, enhancement, illustration and clarification of the results from one method with the results from the other method.
• Development seeks to use the results from one method to help develop or inform the other method, where development is broadly construed to include sampling and implementation, as well as measurement decisions.
• Initiation seeks the discovery of paradox and contradiction, new perspectives of frameworks, the recasting of questions or results from one method with questions or results from the other method.
• Expansion seeks to extend the breadth and range of inquiry by using different methods for different inquiry components (Greene et al., 1989, p. 259).

Of the studies they reviewed, 80 per cent of the primary purposes and half of the 70 total purposes were either complementarity or expansion.

Types of mixed method design

In this section, we consider four common approaches to mixing methods.

Qualitative then quantitative

This design occurs when the findings of the qualitative research are used to develop the quantitative phase of the research. This is a common approach to mixing methods, but one that is sometimes misunderstood. Some primarily quantitative researchers see a limited role for using qualitative research in an exploratory capacity, but always followed by quantitative research. Blalock (1970), for example, considers that 'techniques of participant observation are extremely useful in providing initial insights and hunches that can lead to more careful formulations of the problem and explicit hypotheses', but are rarely sufficient in themselves to stand alone (1970, pp. 45–6). This has led to the perception among some researchers that the qualitative phase of such studies is somehow lesser, not part of the real research so much as paving the way for it. We would see the qualitative phase of such a study as having a developmental purpose in relation to the quantitative phase, and to the study as a whole. Thinking of the different methodological components in terms of their purpose gets away from any suggestion that one is inherently of more value than the other. Even where one method is more prominent, as often may be the case, the use of a properly thought out mixed-method design implies that all the components have a specific purpose and are equally necessary to the overall research.

In the development of a scale to assess and evaluate the learning needs and concerns of prospective parents, Imle and Atwood (1988) attempted to use qualitative and quantitative methods in equal but different ways. They used qualitative methods first, to develop and define concepts that represented the needs and concerns experienced by expectant parents. The inductively generated concepts were then used to develop the Transition to Parenthood Concerns (TPC) Scale. Prospective items were rated for clarity, consistency and content validity by panels of doctoral students and expectant parents before final inclusion in the scale. This is an example of a process designed to meet quantitative psychometric estimates for scale testing while also preserving the meaning of the items from the perspective of expectant parents.

Laurie also used qualitative approaches—interviews and group discussions—in the development of a questionnaire module on the allocation of resources within households, to be included in a large-scale survey of British households.

> Issues and questions emerged from the data collected in the first stage
> of the project which we felt obliged to pursue, not only for
> clarification of the qualitative data but to meet the design imperatives
> of a quantitative, longitudinal study. Without the use of qualitative

methods which allowed the detailed exploration of intra-household resource allocation, it is doubtful that many of these issues would have emerged . . . the use of multiple methods enabled the scope of the questions designed for the BHPS [British Household Panel Study] schedule to be far broader than initially envisaged (Laurie, 1992, p. 165).

Quantitative then qualitative

This approach occurs when the findings of the quantitative research are needed to develop the qualitative phase.

In a three-stage study on juvenile delinquency, Reicher and Emler (1986, cited in Bryman, 1988) initially asked 600 young people, 12 to 15 years old, to complete questionnaire measures of self-reported delinquency and social attitudes. From this, they identified groups which differed sharply in their degree of involvement in delinquency. In the second stage they conducted structured face-to-face interviews with 150 of the original sample about their views on delinquency. The data obtained at this stage formed the basis for an intensive interview study of 60 young people with contrasting levels of involvement in delinquent activities.

Catherine McDonald's (1996) study of the application of neo-institutional theory in the non-profit sector is another example of the use of quantitative research to inform a later stage of qualitative research. (Neo-institutional theory is an approach to organisational analysis that incorporates micro and macro levels of analysis. It 'links micro sociological processes in the form of taken for granted, habituated actions, with macro sociological processes such as the production and maintenance of dominant organisational forms, sectors or fields' (McDonald, 1996, p. 53).) We talk to Catherine about her use of mixed methods later in this chapter.

In both these studies, the quantitative phase was used to identify groups of particular interest that were followed up for more in-depth analysis using qualitative methods. In both this and the qualitative to quantitative design first discussed, the results from one method directly inform the other; what happens in later phases is dependent on the findings from earlier phases.

Qualitative and quantitative concurrently

Mixed qualitative and quantitative designs do not always have to be interdependent to the extent described above. Sometimes quantitative and qualitative components of a study are carried out independently and the conduct of one does not depend on the other. In this case it does not matter whether they are conducted concurrently, sequentially or in any particular order. Different methods may be used to address the same research question, as in a classic triangulation, or relate to different aspects of the research. The purposes of a mixed-method study of this type would generally be triangulation, complementarity or expansion, or some combination of these.

This approach was used by Krahn, Hohn and Kime (1995) in their study of parental experiences of being informed about their child's disability. Interviews about the diagnostic experience were conducted with parents and analysed thematically. Parents also completed quantitative ratings about the professional who informed them of the disability. In this case, different methods were used to obtain different sets of data that together may shed light on how parents experienced the diagnostic process. While parents consistently rated the professionals highly, the interviews revealed considerable dissatisfaction with how the professionals handled the situation. After considering several alternative explanations through statistical means, the researchers concluded that the open-ended interviews both enabled greater nuances of experience to be expressed and encompassed broader aspects of the informing process than the ratings, thus revealing a greater depth and complexity to the informing process than had previously been reported in the literature.

Liz Kelly's (1999) evaluation of a crisis intervention service to follow-up police responses to domestic violence is another example of this approach to mixed methods. Qualitative and quantitative methods were used, for different components of the evaluation brief, and at different stages of the research. As the research progressed, there were various modifications in design, such as rewording some survey questions to reflect current practice terminology, and a follow-up questionnaire to social services agencies was abandoned on the basis of poor response in favour of a smaller number of more targeted telephone interviews. Even so, the methods themselves were not interdependent, in that the findings obtained through one method were not used in the development of another. We talk to Liz later in this chapter about her use of mixed methods in this study and, more generally, in the Child and Woman Abuse Studies Unit at the University of North London.

Mixing qualitative data collection approaches

Just as it is possible to combine quantitative and qualitative methods in order to more thoroughly investigate a research problem, a more thorough understanding of an issue or problem can often be gained from combining a number of qualitative data collection approaches. As with quantitative/qualitative designs, the different approaches may sit side by side or be iterative, with the analysis from one phase forming the basis for the next phase of data collection.

In a study of child welfare workers' understandings of child abuse, Darlington, Osmond and Peile (2001) conducted two rounds of in-depth interviews, followed by focus groups, with twelve child protection workers from the Queensland Department of Families. The study was designed in such a way that each stage was dependent on the previous stage.

In the first interview participants were asked to select and briefly describe a case in which intrafamilial physical abuse was a major issue. The interview then focused on eliciting explanations about how and why the abuse happened, at the case-specific level. Following the first interview, the research team compiled lists of all the explanations that each worker had identified in the first interview, both explicitly and implicitly. Each worker's explanations were presented to them during the second interview and used as a basis for broader discussion of reasons why physical child abuse occurs. The workers were asked to consider a range of alternative contingencies—for example, would the explanation change (and how) if: the mother/father was the identified abuser; the child was younger/older; only one/more children in the family had been abused; there had/had not been other forms of abuse identified; there had/had not been a previous history of abuse, etc. They were also asked to identify any connections or associations between the explanations they had provided. Thus while the first interview concerned a specific case, the second interview encompassed the full range of types of cases with which the worker was involved. In the focus groups the discussion moved to an even more general level, based around a composite list of explanations from all twelve participants.

When findings conflict

Using different methods in the one study always carries the possibility of obtaining contradictory findings. This should not in itself be considered a problem. It is, however, a clear indication that further work may be required to understand better what is happening.

Dorothy Scott (1992) used quantitative and qualitative methods in her study of the role of child health nurses in relation to the social and emotional well-being of mothers of young children (we introduced this study in Chapter 1). Forty-five mothers were interviewed using semi-structured questionnaires and three nurses were observed at work for a week each. The mothers' interviews included a number of structured scales concerned with their attitudes to the nurses' role. In this study, quite different results were obtained through the interviews with mothers and the observations of mother–nurse interaction. The mothers had reported very high levels of acceptance of nurses inquiring about their emotional state and how they were coping with their baby. The nurses, on the other hand, seemed cautious about extending their role to these areas, giving lower acceptability ratings to these items than the mothers. In the observations, however, there was greater congruence with the nurses' responses. Mothers were observed to respond tentatively when nurses initiated discussion of maternal emotional well-being and nurses 'readily retreated to the safer, traditional child-focused issues if the mother seemed to perceive this as intrusive' (1992, p. 352). It is possible that this could have been due to the observer's presence, although the nurses reported that they did not think this was the case, believing that their interactions with the mothers were similar in the absence of the observer.

In this example, the observation of what mothers and nurses *did* provided additional data that challenged the findings from the interviews. The observational data indicated the issue was much more interactional than was evident from the mothers' interviews alone, with the nurses seeming to retreat at signs of maternal discomfort.

The discrepancy in the data was in this case not a problem

in itself. Rather, the methods 'measured' different things. The semi-structured interviews measured the mothers' attitudinal norms while the observational data measured the behavioural norms which appeared to govern nurse–mother interaction. Whether, as here, explanations can be found, or whether one needs to go back to the field and look again, discrepant findings can be a catalyst to carrying an analysis and understanding forward and, as such, are best regarded as an opportunity rather than a constraint. Bryman's view is that discrepancies in the data should be expected; what matters is how one responds to them:

> Discrepancies between the findings deriving from research in which quantitative and qualitative research are combined are not in the least unusual. Further, it is in the spirit of the idea of triangulation that inconsistent results may emerge; it is not in its spirit that one should simply opt for one set of findings rather than another. Discrepancies may also prompt the researcher to probe certain issues in greater depth, which may lead to fruitful areas of inquiry in their own right (Bryman, 1988, p. 134).

Stories from the field

We include here three inside stories about the use of mixed methods. First, Liz Kelly talks about her evaluation of a program to implement a crisis intervention service to follow-up police responses to domestic violence in the UK. Catherine McDonald then talks about her use of mixed methods in her study of non-profit human service organisations and, finally, Cheryl Tilse talks about her use of a combination of qualitative approaches in her study of older people who had placed their spouse in a nursing home.

Liz Kelly—Domestic violence matters

We talked with Liz Kelly about the evaluation she and her colleagues at the Child and Woman Abuse Studies Unit, University of North London, did on Domestic Violence Matters—a program to implement a crisis intervention service to follow-up police responses to domestic violence. It is a complex program with three discrete aims, each of which had to be evaluated in terms of both outcome and process. The study is published as *Domestic Violence Matters*

(1999) by the Home Office. Liz and her colleagues used both qualitative and quantitative methods to address different aspects of the
three strands of the program. Liz is absolutely clear that neither
approach is privileged, that both are equally important to the
research. She talks here about her use of mixed methods.

Liz: *Domestic Violence Matters* was the most complicated
          piece of research I have ever done . . . the project had
          three discrete aims. One was to deliver crisis inter-
          vention by civilians after police intervention to anyone
          calling about domestic violence. The second was to
          increase a law enforcement response and the third
          was to develop inter-agency work in the local areas.
          There was no simple way of addressing all those
          things, and [they wanted] a process evaluation as well
          . . . So each of those strands was addressed through
          multi-methodological strategies. The crisis intervention
          was addressed through having a database that the
          workers filled in, and then a detailed questionnaire to
          all the women who used the service, and interviews
          with the workers delivering the service. I would also
          just pop in and hang around or I would go to collect
          data and hang around for longer and I would go to
          their canteen and chat with the workers and so I got a
          feel of [how they were] doing the work, and I did that
          at different times in the day and sometimes in the
          evening.
              The police strand involved three much shorter
          questionnaires at timed intervals at the beginning of
          the project, in the middle, and towards the end, to try
          and see whether there was a shift in understanding
          around domestic violence being a crime and police
          responses. We also tried to get actual operational data
          from the police about the number of arrests and about
          the outcomes of the cases, and again I hung around
          and observed the police officers, particularly those in
          the specialist unit who were supposed to deal with
          domestic violence . . . Then towards the end I did two
          focus groups with police officers to explore with them
          some of the questions that had come up about ways
          that the ambitions of the project hadn't been realised

and how they would explain it, what they thought about it and what ideas they had about how it could have been done differently. Then with the inter-agency, we initially sent a questionnaire to 200 voluntary agencies but we didn't get a very good return—that was supposed to be a two-stage questionnaire, one at the beginning and one towards the end again to look at change and contact with the project and we decided that instead of doing that, we would do telephone interviews with 20 or 30 agencies that the project had had the most contact with.

Using mixed methods

We asked Liz to elaborate on one of the strands of the project in more detail, to show how the methods interrelated and what each brought to the evaluation.

Liz: Okay, let's talk about the crisis intervention. It couldn't just rely on the database. What the database would tell us was, how many women, did [the response] happen within 24 hours, as it was supposed to, which other agencies they were referred on to, and how many times subsequently they were in contact with the project. That's basic information, but it doesn't tell you much about the process. It doesn't tell you whether it made a difference to women, how or in what way. They are the kind of benchmarking performance things that people measure, but those measures tell you they performed at that level—they don't tell you anything about the quality of the work and what impact it had on anybody.

It couldn't just rely on talking to the workers, or even observing the workers, because they are obviously going to want to believe that their work has an impact, as they should; and they are going to know what their interaction was, but they are not going to know what that meant to the person they were interacting with. And also I think they didn't necessarily have an overview. They didn't work with cases as a caseworker. Because it was crisis intervention it had to be whoever was there. You would respond to what comes in, so they wouldn't have the sense necessarily of the process for any individual woman, and I think sometimes they were so busy, they didn't use the database as a way of having a sense of what is happening to this woman over time. They were just responding to what was happening in the immediacy of the situation. Other times when they had less workload, they were more able to do that. The workers wouldn't know whether any of the referrals they made were taken up, whether they were useful; and they would probably have most information on the cases where the model worked best, so the women for whom this model worked, who used the project, those would be the cases that they would know.

So we had to have feedback from the users, but we also had to have it in a way that was manageable for us and doable, given that there were over 1000 users of this project over three years. The idea of doing in-depth interviews with that number is just impossible, and also you can't analyse that amount of data. So there are practicalities involved, and we had to use a method that didn't require so much of our time and didn't require enormous amounts of time for analysis, so we used a questionnaire. Within that questionnaire there was a lot of space for qualitative information, but not collected in the traditional way qualitative data tends to be thought of. There were very few forced-choice questions, [other than] did the police come, how long did it take them to come, etc. And then there was a question, how would you describe the responses of the police to you—did they do anything that was particularly useful, if so what was it, did they do something that wasn't helpful, if so what was it. And then the same kinds of questions for the support workers . . . When we asked them what was helpful, and what made a difference to them, it wasn't all the things that people want to measure. It was really fundamental things: that the workers named violence; that they were really clear that it wasn't the women's fault; being confronted with the fact that men chose to be violent, which wasn't the explanation that the women were currently using themselves . . .

What I think is interesting about that was that we wouldn't have found that out it if we hadn't had the open-ended questions in the questionnaire, but also, I think it wouldn't have been as powerful if we had done 20 or 30 in-depth interviews. What we had was 230 questionnaires where a really significant proportion of respondents were saying the same thing.

Liz also commented generally on the use of mixed methods at the Child and Woman Abuse Studies Unit.

Liz: I began as a qualitative researcher and then the second research grant we got here was to do an exploratory prevalence study of sexual abuse. That obviously had to be a quantitative study on some level and so we needed a staff member who had that expertise because I didn't, and that person, Linda Regan, has been here ever since, and so in a way it's the linking of both our skills.

But equally, I think it's about her understanding the importance of meaning, and me understanding the importance of numbers if you are talking about influencing policy-makers. But also, the importance of being able to ascertain whether things really are in the data or not, because while I absolutely accept that we bring our subjectivity and subjective meanings to the work that we are doing, at the same time I think we need to be rigorous about whether things are there or not. We had this really interesting experience in the prevalence study where three of us coded 1244 questionnaires and we ended up with perceptions about what we thought was in the data and actually it wasn't there to the extent that we thought it was. We thought that there was much more abuse by brothers and we didn't think there was as much abuse by uncles—it was about what we noticed, what resonated with us, and actually that isn't always [what the data are

131

saying] . . . given that we work in an area where there is a possibility that what we say, what we conclude, might influence policy and, if it does, that has a direct impact on the lives of women and children, I feel we have a responsibility to be careful . . . The other side of that I think is a more realistic position. We have never hidden the fact that we are feminists, but I think that does mean that you are held to account and to accusations of bias in a way that people who pretend a neutral position are not, so one of the ways we have responded to that is to never publish anything where we weren't really certain that it was actually in the data, so that we can defend the position from the research material and not an ideological position.

Yvonne: And mixed methods have been an effective means of doing that?

Yes. I think it gives you a kind of discipline, that actually counting how many think or say a particular thing matters, and the kind of discipline of paying attention to what people are actually telling you . . . And then the qualitative for me is, okay, how do you make sense of some of these things, what do they mean, what is the complexity of them, because life is always more messy than tick boxes.

Liz also talked about the advantage of mixed methods from research participants' points of view, suggesting that different people may prefer to provide information about themselves in different ways.

Liz: I think the thing about questionnaires that is very interesting is that they automatically give confidentiality in a way that participant observation or interviews don't. With interviews, researchers have to talk through with participants how they will disguise their identity, include this or exclude that. Whereas with a questionnaire it's very clear—we are not asking for your name. I have a suspicion that for some people, not everybody, but for some people that gives them a kind of freedom to say things, a kind of security about the fact that it is confidential, so they reveal things . . . So that led me to think, actually, we can be incredibly arrogant and presumptive about our ability to make a context where it is safe to talk about these things in like five minutes, ten minutes, whatever it might be, and that maybe we need to think about people as complicated, that there is no perfect method, so there will be some for whom the questionnaire is a much easier thing to do, is a much easier form of communication in which to tell complicated difficult things, and there will be other people for whom spoken communication is easier. And then if we start talking about women and children with disabilities, we enter another whole realm again, so I think about mixed methods as enabling different kinds of telling.

Catherine McDonald—Institutionalised organisations?

Catherine McDonald used a combination of quantitative and qualitative methods for her PhD study on the application of neo-institutional organisational theory to non-profit organisations in Queensland. She has subsequently reported on methodological issues in relation to this study (McDonald, 1997, 1999).

The research was conducted in two stages. Stage one involved a survey of 500 non-profit services, from which twelve services with either very high or very low organisational commitment were identified. Catherine then sought to test each of the propositions of neo-institutional theory in each of these services. She did this through semi-structured interviews with the CEO and with one worker directly involved with clients, and through analysis of public documents on the goals and financial status of each of the organisations.

We were particularly interested in Catherine's rationale for using mixed methods and the way she combined them in this study.

Why mixed methods?

> *Catherine:* The reason that it went to a mixed-method type approach was [actually] two reasons. One was because I was looking at a whole field of organisa-tions, so one approach could never deal with the

complexity of the social phenomenon that I was examining . . . you have to come at it from lots of different angles to get a fix on it. The other reason was that the body of theory itself invoked different levels of analysis so you had to develop a methodology that worked at those different levels of analysis. So that led me to mixed methods almost inevitably. In mixed-methods work most people go qualitative, then quantitative and back to qualitative. I went quantitative to qualitative. What I wanted to do was get a feel for the whole series of organisations on a key variable and then pick out organisations where I could go and look at stuff in-depth. So where they varied on the one variable a lot, they were obviously key organisations for saying where these sorts of processes that I was talking about were either being enacted or not being enacted. This means you could get a real fix on the theory . . . I started off with a key variable in all of this, organisational commitment, because nearly all of the literature around non-profits argues that these people are highly committed . . . Organisational commitment itself is a fairly complex variable and there are a lot of dimensions to it, but there has been a lot of work done about developing what the concept actually is, the component parts of the concept, and then developing instruments that pick up all the component parts . . . So I thought, right, there is a whole body of theory saying what that variable actually consists of. There are excellent instruments developed . . . It would be silly not to use that key variable to try and denote the sites where some qualitative work would make some sense.

The survey

Catherine: I had to spend a lot of time in the first place constructing a sample frame . . . You can never find all
the organisations and there's no one list of them
anywhere . . . So I constructed a sample frame from
about three or four different sources . . . [there were]

about 1200 organisations in it . . . Then I did a random
sample out of that, sent off about 500 questionnaires
and ended up with a return rate of about 50 per cent.
What I wanted that for was to find outliers and
find people with a high organisational commitment
and those with low organisational commitment. And
they became the sites for me to go and do further
work, drawing on a model from neo-institutional
theory. And that was a complex model in itself. It
was eight propositions of why these organisations
were what we would call highly institutionalised
and therefore considered to be different . . . But I then
had to go and actually talk to people in those organisations about the sorts of things that the theory said
would be happening. If it was a highly institutionalised
organisation, there would be values congruence.
There was a whole series of things. One of them
was evaluation—normal processes of inspection and
evaluation would be suspended. They were. In highly
institutionalised organisations there was virtually no
internal inspection. It was just all taken for granted
that everything would be okay.

The interviews

Catherine: It was 24 interviews all up. There were about eight
organisations which had scored very low on the
organisational commitment and the rest were in the
upper ranks . . . So I took the very highest and the very
lowest and went off and had a look at them. And it
was just what the theory said would happen. So in
the high-commitment organisations the theory was
absolutely validated. All the propositions, all the things
that I said I would observe there, I observed. And in
the low ones, all the opposite things were there. The
theory fitted like a glove . . .
They were semi-structured interviews and pretty
in-depth because what I was actually doing was
getting them to talk about their organisation and really
getting them to reveal how they constructed that

organisation. And they raved—each interview was an hour-and-a-half to two hours long.

The document analysis

Catherine: I also used organisational records to look at some of the propositions . . . I wanted to have a look at all their aims and objectives because one of the things the theory said is that the organisation's aims and objectives, its goals, would be so broadly stated that they were completely untestable. You know, things like 'this organisation has been formed to save children'. I also wanted to have a look at their financial records because one of the other things that the theory said is that certain patterns of financial dependence on external constituents means that they have to conform to the expectations of those constituents. So I needed to look at their ratios of financial dependence which meant looking at accounts . . . With the goals stuff, that was just a content analysis, looking at the sorts of goals and things they said about themselves and the financial stuff was just really simple sums . . .

Yvonne: So you did the survey, then the interviews and then the content analysis, which sounds as though it included a combination qualitative and quantitative analysis.

Catherine: That was it. What I was doing was building a composite picture. I had eight propositions of what these organisations should be doing and not all of them were amenable to a single analytical technique or methodological data-gathering technique. They all needed different ones . . . You've got this phenomenon that has got many different characteristics and you need multiple ways of getting at it so you're building a credible composite picture. You've got to get enough of the different types of data to build the picture and each of them have to be conceptually congruent, so there's got to be an overarching theory or framework that hangs it all together, and I think that's the trick with mixed methods. If you don't have

that overarching analytical framework that puts it all together, then you've just got a pastiche.

Yvonne: There's also something about your purpose, isn't there, because you're very clear that the purpose of the survey was to identify organisations for the next stage so you could argue in a sense that this was to get to the point where you could use the theory?

Catherine: Yes, that's right—to really test out whether it was a living and breathing theory. People often do it the other way around, like they do qualitative work so they can go and determine what the key concepts are and can then do quantitative work by using instruments that measure what they're looking at. I had the theory first and I was going from the theory down into the field. A lot of people start in the field, find the theory—use the qualitative, find what the important constructs are and the central relationships between them, which then hopefully would lead them to a body of theory from which they can then construct their quantitative work. So it depends which way you're going, how you do it.

Yvonne: Without the quantitative stage, you would have had to do considerable prior qualitative work to try to identify the services inductively, before you could start to test the theory. The survey enabled you to use the construct of organisational commitment to find the services quite quickly, so you could then commence the qualitative research at a theory testing stage.

Catherine: Yes, it's a real shortcut. I just don't know how I would have done it otherwise. I would have had to do an awful lot more than 24 interviews, which was not possible . . . And I'd never really know that I was sampling right and that's the whole bedevilment when you're doing theory testing. It's a very different way of using qualitative work. One of the things that became clearer and clearer to me was that this was essentially a positivist model. I was using qualitative work within a positivist framework.

Potential pitfalls in mixing methods

Yvonne: What are the pitfalls with mixed methods?

Catherine: That one bit won't speak to the other. I think that's really it—that they have no linkage. No, the other pitfall from a research point of view is that you're jack of all trades and master of none and so that's pretty scary . . . [You] can never be expert in all of them. Theoretically I suppose what you should do is gather around you experts in those various methods and direct them, but most people don't have the opportunity for that. So if you're going to use mixed methods I guess keep it as simple as possible, keep the analytical methods that you're using as simple as possible otherwise you're going to get out of your depth pretty quickly in the analysis.

Cheryl Tilse—The long goodbye

Cheryl's use of observation (Chapter 4) was just one of the data-collection approaches she used in her study of visiting practices in nursing homes. She also conducted in-depth interviews and analysed documents. She is very clear that no one method would have enabled as full an understanding of the visiting experience as she achieved with the combination of data-collection approaches. She is talking here about what each of the methods brought to the study.

Yvonne: What kinds of things did you pick up from having multiple data collection methods that you wouldn't have picked up from one alone?

Cheryl: I interviewed the spouses first so I came in with a perspective of the spouses and an understanding of what the purpose and meaning of visiting for them was. That was important in how it situated me. I got lots from the two methods that I wouldn't have got from just watching. From just watching I couldn't get who [the staff] saw as difficult and why they were seen as difficult and how the staff understood the purpose and meaning of visiting, of why families visited. But if

I hadn't had the observations I wouldn't have been able to pick up the use of space, the way people were approached, how impossible it was to talk to other people when they were sitting down the end of the verandah with a spouse who couldn't speak . . . I could actually see how lonely visiting in a congregate setting could be, which made me understand that much better. The observation was also important to me because I actually situated myself as a visitor, so I've reflected on my own experience of whether I was welcomed, whether I was introduced to people, whether I was given a cup of tea when the tea trolley went by or whether I was ignored.

Yvonne: With those different methods and the analysis, I'm interested in the relative importance of each to the final product. How did they feed into each other at the end?

Cheryl: I suppose the most important part of the final product was the perspective of the older spouses. I really wanted them to be central because in the final analysis it was really about them and what it meant to them and then the context in which they visited . . . The main things that came out were in the interviews with the spouses and the observations. The interviews with staff confirmed and supported things but they weren't strong enough to stand alone.

Yvonne: Could you have done it just with the in-depth interviews and the observations?

Cheryl: I think it would have been a weakened methodology. If I had just done the observations there's a risk that I would have had no staff perspective. I'm just observing and I'm identifying strongly with these older people, but the fact that I also talked to staff showed me that it wasn't the 'terrible staff'—I'd listened to families but staff understood the situation differently, and without talking to them, you couldn't actually understand that. You could just observe they don't listen to people. All their signals are 'We don't have time for you' and yet when you talked to them it came across as something quite different. So I think [mixing methods] enhanced the complexity of understanding, of saying it's not 'good guys' and 'bad guys' here. It's people not understanding what the issues are for each other. I think also that the observations would be weaker standing alone because it would be harder to observe if you didn't talk to staff, if you didn't value their views, to come in as a researcher and say I'm interested in visitors—I've got no interest in your life other than that this is where you work. I thought I'd have a lot of resistance to interviews, but in fact the staff really liked being interviewed. Nobody talked to them much about their work or their perspective on things. And some of them had very practical and good ideas of what they'd like to do but felt constrained by their workload or by the attitude of [senior staff]. So I think [without the staff interviews] the observations would have been harder to do and I would have understood less.

Comments

Mixing methods is an increasingly common approach to research. Whatever epistemological concerns researchers may have, in practical terms it makes good sense. Real-world research questions, by their very nature, tend to be complex and very often require a range of research approaches in order to answer them adequately. In this chapter's stories, Liz Kelly and Catherine McDonald have explained their rationale for using both quantitative and qualitative methods. Cheryl Tilse provided an equally clear rationale for the combination of qualitative approaches that she used, convinced that no one approach would have yielded the depth and range of understanding possible with a mixed approach.

Just as 'eclectic' counselling practice, when clearly thought through and purposeful, can respond to complex needs more adequately than any one approach on its own, a mixed-methods approach to research also has this potential. An important key though is the need to be clear about which approaches are being used, what the purpose and intended outcome of each is, and how they interrelate. While complex problems can be responded to and investigated more adequately, the risk in letting go of specialisation is that research skills will become too thinly spread, potentially reducing the benefit of the approach. We need to aim for increased breadth of response options without diminishing the depth of skills. This can be addressed by working in teams with qualitative and quantitative specialists. In Liz Kelly's team, this works well because of an underlying appreciation of the worth of both approaches and of the strengths of each of the team members, as well as a common purpose in advancing understanding and the alleviation of violence against women and children.

In the following chapter, we leave data collection to focus on the next stage of research, data analysis.

7

Analysing data

There are many ways to do qualitative analysis. Tesch (1990) identified over twenty separate approaches that between them encompass a broad range of methodologies and epistemological perspectives. There are also many texts providing detailed guides to the practicalities of doing qualitative data analysis (see, for example, Glaser & Strauss, 1967; Strauss, 1987; Dey, 1993; Miles & Huberman, 1994; Lofland & Lofland, 1995; Strauss & Corbin, 1998; Taylor & Bogdan, 1998). In this chapter we have opted to avoid 'potted versions' of research methodologies and restating analysis techniques that are readily available elsewhere.

While there are many different approaches to qualitative data analysis, in practice most approaches involve similar stages. Whatever the research purpose and question, certain analytic choices have to be made—what data to collect, from whom, how to focus the analysis and how to structure the research report.

Data for analysis may come from many sources and be in many forms. They may be obtained through interviews, observation, or content analysis of existing materials, and may include interview tapes or transcripts, observation field notes, notes on interview context and process, analytic notes and memos, or journal entries. The level and extent of analysis of data from the various sources will depend on the purpose for which the data was collected and involves choices that need to be made for each project.

While we do not hold firmly to any one way of doing data analysis, we are absolutely clear of the need to be as explicit as possible about what is being done and why. Taylor and Bogdan (1998) suggest that all qualitative research reports should 'provide enough information about how your research was conducted to enable readers to discount your account or to understand it in the context of how it was produced' (1988, p. 168).

The following section focuses on some key stages of qualitative data analysis. Our comments are particularly relevant to approaches that seek to identify themes or patterns in the data. These include studies that are conducted inductively, with a view to generating new theory, as well as those to test an existing theory which use a more deductive approach. This is followed by the presentation of some perspectives on data analysis from four of our researchers: Catherine McDonald uses a deductive approach to analysis, testing the applicability of neo-institutional theory to the non-profit organisations she studied, while the approaches used by Cheryl Tilse, Anne Coleman and Caroline Thomas are essentially inductive.

Transcribing

Most researchers would agree that any audio-recorded data that are to be systematically analysed will need to be transcribed. Transcribing is a time-consuming process, especially for researchers who lack the resources to employ a transcriber. Estimates of the time it takes to transcribe an hour of tape vary according to the level of detail required for the transcripts, the quality of the tape, and the number of voices on the tape. A reasonably good quality recording, with an interviewer and one respondent, transcribed at a general level of detail by a proficient transcriber with a transcribing machine, will take around three hours per hour of tape.

For most qualitative research, transcription at a general level of detail would include, at a minimum, identification of long pauses (with the number of seconds or minutes typed in) and bracketed indications of obvious emotional content such as laughing, crying or sighing. There will inevitably be a great deal of contextual material that does not get onto the tape, including non-verbals and aspects of the interview setting that may impact on what is said and how. The researcher's field notes can provide at least one perspective on these issues and thus should be sufficiently comprehensive to include any contextual factors that may have a bearing on the research.

Some specialised forms of analysis, such as conversation analysis (Psathas, 1995), narrative analysis (Riessman, 1993), or discourse analysis (Gee, 1999), may require more detailed transcription. Riessman recommends a more general transcription of the entire interview and then retranscription for detailed analysis of sections of particular interest. Gee on the other hand suggests 'transcribing for more detail than may in the end be relevant' (1999, p. 88).

Wherever possible, be prepared to pay for an experienced transcriber, who should be well briefed about the level of detail required. This will vary from study to study and from researcher to researcher. It is also important to decide a process for dealing with words or phrases the transcriber cannot hear or is unfamiliar with. We suggest identifying such places in the transcript with an agreed symbol such as a series of crosses or question marks, and having an understanding that the transcriber will not try to guess. Experienced transcribers will understand the importance of confidentiality, but it is essential to address this issue specifically with each job.

Transcribing is not only a specialised technical skill, it can also be hard work emotionally. Where sensitive topics are raised in interviews, be prepared to spend time to allow the transcriber to talk about their emotional response to the transcripts (see Matocha, 1992). For the transcriber, the powerful emotions experienced can be particularly intense, undistilled by other aspects of the interview and the research context.

Becoming familiar with the data

Once the transcript has been checked for accuracy, listening to the tape again, with the transcript in hand, can be an invaluable way of getting a fuller sense of what the text is about. It is difficult to obtain a good sense of familiarity with the data during in-depth interviews or while observing, as there are so many other things to attend to during data collection. While the researcher undoubtedly forms overall impressions, there is no substitute for this next stage of immersing oneself in the data. For Riessman (1993), 'A focus for analysis often emerges, or becomes clearer, as I see what respondents say' at this stage (1993, p. 57).

Coding

Coding is the process of creating categories and assigning them to selected data (Dey, 1993). In qualitative research this process is sometimes referred to as indexing (Mason, 1996). While coding is a term used in both quantitative and qualitative research, very different processes are involved. In quantitative research, coding is part of data management and involves numerically transforming the data in preparation for analysis. In qualitative research, coding is an integral part of the analysis, involving sifting through the data, making sense of it and categorising it in various ways. The analytic choices made here about what to code and how will influence every stage of the research from here on.

Qualitative analysis is generally concerned with identifying patterns in the data—different ways in which the data relate to each other. The kinds of patterns identified depend very much on the focus of the study. Lofland and Lofland (1995), for example, have identified a number of levels at which analysis can be focused. These may range from the microscopic to the macroscopic and may be social practices, episodes, encounters, roles, relationships, groups, settlements, social worlds, lifestyles or subcultures. Within each, the specific aspect of focus may be cognitive meanings, feelings or inequalities, and any given study may be focused at one or more levels and one or more aspects. They stress that this approach is meant to provide a mindset for coding that 'should provide you a general orientation to the *kinds of things* for which to look in coding data, *not* a preformed schemata of things for which to code' (1995, p. 122). Bogdan and Biklen (1992) also present a useful list of possible kinds of codes to develop and likewise stress that they are meant to assist in categorising data and not to be rigidly adhered to. Their list includes setting/context codes, definition of the situation codes, perspectives held by participants, participants' ways of thinking about people and objects, process codes, activity codes, event codes, strategy codes, relationship and social structure codes, and methods codes. Again, a study may focus on just one or a number of these types of codes.

Lists such as these are helpful in so far as they draw attention to the vast array of possible ways to focus analysis. They open up the possibilities but also make the need to focus abundantly clear—no one study can hope to look at everything. The danger is that they may provide a false sense of security, a belief that a focus for analysis will emerge at some stage. In practice, decisions about the levels of analysis and types of codes should flow from the research purpose and question, and so be made early on—data collection, too, ought to have been focused in such a way as to obtain the kind of data that will enable the research question to be answered. This approach does not predetermine what themes will emerge but certainly shapes the kinds of themes. For example, Yvonne Darlington's (1996) study of sexually abused women was primarily concerned with women's subjective experience of the impact of childhood sexual abuse in their lives. In keeping with this phenomenological focus, the interview transcripts were coded with a particular view to relationships and experienced emotions.

Even so, too tight a focus on particular types of data at an early stage of analysis carries the risk that unexpected and unanticipated relationships between the data will be missed. We suggest trying a number of different ways of looking at the data, including looking for differences as well as similarities.

Coding in a team

While coding in a team is essentially no different to coding alone, the processes have to be very explicit and consistently applied. While team coding can be a powerful motivator for rigour, if done poorly the potential for comprising both reliability and validity is multiplied.

Team coding worked well on a study on understanding hope in mental illness (Darlington & Bland, 1999), where both authors coded. We both coded the first few interviews in each of three data sets (consumers, family members and workers), and through this developed our code book. Once we were confident of our own and each other's coding, we divided the remaining interviews between us but still cross-coded a selection of each other's work. Discussions about difficult or unclear coding decisions were invaluable, stopping to ask questions like: Does this bit fit in a category we already have or is it really a new category, something we haven't come across before? Does it require a new code? Having to argue for any new code to a fellow researcher proved to be a good test of whether it was really needed.

Fielding and Lee found numerous instances of differences among team members getting in the way of completing qualitative analysis, but also note the potential of teamwork to enhance qualitative research:

> [Team research] obliges researchers to be more explicit about their assumptions and particular understandings of qualitative research.

Team research makes the research process more transparent. Working in teams might help to counteract other pathologies, such as the unchecked proliferation of codes and the contrasting problem of coding which is too 'thin' or superficial (Fielding & Lee, 1998, p. 119).

Do I need a computer program?

The answer to the question of whether a particular piece of research requires a computer program will always be in the first instance, 'maybe'. It will depend on the amount of data and what is to be done with it. There is no doubt that computer programs to assist qualitative data analysis can be of enormous benefit, particularly for studies where there are large amounts of data. A computer program can manage amounts of data that it would be impossible for any researcher to keep in their head and, at the same time, retrieve, or bring to the fore, selected parts of the data for detailed analysis. There is a potential downside to this, in that the capability of the program may encourage sloppy data management early on— coding anything and everything 'just in case', or justifying very broad codes on the basis that one can come back later and refine the coding system if need be. While this can be an advantage in that closure is not reached too early on, the risks are that this can be mistaken for the analytical work integral to coding and that, after a lot of work, one is no closer to understanding what the data mean.

There are an ever-increasing number and variety of programs available, thus knowing what you want a program to do is very important. The two types currently most commonly used in qualitative analysis are code and retrieve programs and theory building programs (Fielding & Lee, 1998; Grbich, 1999). It is important to choose a program that will support rather than constrain your analysis. The availability of training and/or ongoing technical assistance is also an important consideration.

Stories from the field

In this chapter, our stories are relatively brief excerpts from the interviews with some of the researchers introduced earlier. These are not intended to provide comprehensive coverage of the possible approaches to qualitative data analysis or of all the stages in the analysis process—that would require a book in itself. The array of approaches presented here is indicative of the complexity of the field and of the need for researchers to make choices about data analysis (as with every stage of the research process) in the context of the particular project. We have included excerpts from our interviews with Cheryl Tilse, Anne Coleman, Catherine McDonald and Caroline Thomas.

Cheryl Tilse—The long goodbye

Here Cheryl talks about transcribing in-depth interviews and analysing the data from the interviews, the observations and the nursing home documentation.

Transcribing

Cheryl: I had one person who is an experienced transcriber transcribe the interviews in *The Ethnograph* [computer program] format. So the prime tool to help the analysis was to have the interviews transcribed in absolute detail. I asked the transcriber to put in brackets, pauses, crying, that sort of thing but it wasn't the very fine detailed transcribing of conversational analysis. It was very much 'type down what they say' . . .

Yvonne: How important is it to have a good transcriber and a good relationship with your transcriber?

Cheryl: I think it's really important. I thought it was also really important that the same person did them all because she knew what I was talking about and she knew the study and she knew what I was trying to do. It was really important to say things like, 'Don't guess. It's not about that. It's about you typing them up for me and just tell me what's not clear and then it's my job to make the thing perfect. I will go back and check it.' It was also good that I had a good relationship with her in that she got very distressed—I mean they're really sad tapes, they're all about grief and loss and people crying—and I could say to her, 'How are you doing with this stuff?' because I found when I re-listened to the tapes it was actually more upsetting than when I was doing the interview. When you heard just how profoundly unhappy some people were, it was very moving and I thought, 'She sits at home typing this' . . . So it was really important to give her a chance to debrief or say, 'Well, how do you go when it's so sad? I find them really sad.' We did a lot of this by telephone and she'd say, 'I get up and walk around the kitchen, have a bit of a cry and go back to it.' So, I think it was important that somebody was really listening to what they were typing and really trying to get it down. It wasn't a simple typing job.

Analysing the in-depth interviews

Cheryl: I had mounds of transcripts—very long interviews. I suppose I was always very clear that *The Ethnograph* was just a cut-and-paste tool and that I was doing the analysis. I just did the usual process of coding line by line into categories . . . trying to code as I went along so it was a developing process, rather than say, 'Here's all the interviews, now I'll sit down and code them.' I did a couple of interviews and got them transcribed and coded them and kept working on the general themes. I kept a code book and so if in Interview 3 I introduced a new code, I would go back to Interview 1 and say, 'Is it there called something else?' so that I didn't actually introduce a code in Interview 10 that I hadn't checked all the other interviews for. That was really important—because you suddenly got a sense of 'I'm calling it something else in the early stages but the more I understand what it is I can code it slightly differently, so I need to find those codes'. *The Ethnograph* was handy because you could add things together and do things like that . . . I took four interviews and then I wrote them up as if it was going to be a chapter on four interviews— here are the common themes; here are quotes that support these themes; here are the differences. And then when I'd done eight, I wrote the chapter again on eight interviews. I was trying to see what was staying in as common themes or what was dropping out, so I really kept on top of the analysis . . . I did four big versions . . . It was a really good way for me to stay on top of such a mound of material and feel that I was writing about it all the time. The other thing I did was use the face sheet option [in *The Ethnograph*] for separating out the themes. The things I looked for were gender, dementia and non-dementia, because the literature says that the spouse with dementia is a much more traumatic care-giving situation than a spouse who has a physical disability. I also looked at age groups . . . to say, 'Well, do they differ?' If I re-analyse it and say. 'Well, I'm looking at it this way, how do these themes come out?', *The Ethnograph* was very useful for doing that—for grouping and seeing the differences . . .

When I saw a common theme I'd take that theme and then say, 'If it's a common theme then I have to find it in every interview'. Or I'd identify which interviews did not reflect the theme. So I was constantly trying to keep in this view, that there might be some people who didn't fit and I'm not just selecting the same four or five interviews that are very rich [data]. I wanted to have an example from each interview and then I could write it down . . . but what I did in the final draft was actually select out the examples that encapsulated the theme best. But the process of analysis was making sure that I said it was common because it was common . . . And when I knew who it wasn't common with, I addressed that in the next chapter . . . So I ended up with another chapter on difference and divergence and that's where I look at men and women and [other differences]. But I also then talked about three people who really didn't fit, which was almost like case study reporting and saying 'this one man is hardly quoted . . . I was determined not to leave him out but it was very clear he didn't fit in'.

Analysing the observational data

Cheryl: What I did here was try and sort through the observations. I was trying to link them to themes of inclusion
and exclusion and so I really looked at them in those
terms rather than just describing this happened to this
visitor, this happened to that visitor—I looked at them
all and said, 'Well, what practices and provisions
included people and what excluded family visitors?'
So I tried to structure it that way so it allowed me to
contain heaps of information—notebooks of descriptions of what happened to people. I had some basic
research questions, for example, 'How were they
provided for?' So I did a description of what the provision was—were there family visiting rooms? Were
there kettles? Was there equipment for families, notebooks for families to write things in? So I looked at
provision and then I looked at the treatment of visitors
and when I talked about treatment it was just this
theme of inclusion/exclusion.

The document analysis

Cheryl: The content analysis basically just picked up what
guides [the nursing homes] had—they'd have some
guides to family visiting or notes for families. Then I
did a content analysis and identified what roles they
constructed for families—are they resources? Like,
'We appreciate your help with feeding and bringing
clothes', or are they seen as, 'Come join us. You're
part of the family. We'd like to get to know you.' You
know, the underlying themes. So it was really interesting, seeing how particular facilities constructed very
clear roles [for families].

Anne Coleman—Five star motels

Anne talks here about her thematic analysis of the data from her
observations and informal interviews for her research with homeless

people (Coleman, 2001), and about her use of *The Ethnograph* program for managing text-based data (Seidel 1998).

Analysing the observational data

Anne: In Phase One [observation] I colour-coded everything. I was really only interested in three things—people, spaces and what they were doing in the spaces. So I took the computer notes that I'd typed from the original field notes and I went through every page of those notes with three coloured highlighters—green for spaces, orange for people and purple for acts—and every space named, every person, group, member of a group, whatever, I colour-highlighted the whole lot. I'm fairly visual so once I got it to this stage it was easy. It made sense to me because I'd never keep all that together in my head. And the journal—I didn't do much analysis on the journal because in a sense it was an analysis of what I was feeling that day and what I was thinking and it was also a record of why I'd gone one way methodologically and not the other. It was used all the way through in the final write-up as a way of illustrating, or making a point, or putting a date on something, but it wasn't analysed and used in that sense . . .

In Phase Two [informal interviews] I repeated the way I'd recorded the observations in Phase One so that any time I wasn't directly engaging with people or following that up I'd be having a bit of a sit and writing down what I'd seen. So that was an identical process. I didn't want to record those conversations because I knew they were brief and I was going to have most of them on the run, for example, 'I'm from Queensland University, I'm interested in this, do you come to the Valley often? Have you got five minutes to chat?' And that's all it would be. I'd have the conversation and then I'd run away and write some memory-dot points, this is this, this and this. The only exception was if somebody had said something in a way that was just so brilliant or so clever or just 'I wish

I'd said that', then I would write that down. I repeated the process of typing the [handwritten] field notes into the field notes computer format. I'd go home and from those dot point notes write up the conversation as a separate conversation . . . and again the analysis of that was basically thematic. What I was looking for was the breadth of the range of opinions, so I would have been really disappointed if everybody had said exactly the same thing—they didn't of course.

Using *The Ethnograph* to order the data from the in-depth interviews

Anne: I like to hold something in my hand while I'm reading it and I was extremely concerned about whether using *The Ethnograph* would somehow take the life out of the conversation or transform the information in some way, but I used it partly because I wanted to learn it and this was the perfect opportunity, and the other thing that it was really useful for was as a management tool. Although it was really useful, I've got to say I kept going back to the transcripts, to the hand-held ones. And I did a lot of stuff by hand . . . I did the initial couple of rounds of coding by hand. When I thought I had a broad enough idea about the whole length and breadth of the content and I wasn't coding myself in too tightly, I then entered them in *The Ethnograph* and got all the numbered lines and started to pull the themes out there. But I never totally relied on *The Ethnograph*. To me, it was a management tool.

Catherine McDonald—Institutionalised organisations?

Here Catherine talks about how she analysed the in-depth interviews for her study on the application of neo-institutional theory to the non-profit sector in Queensland. Catherine's work is an example of a very structured approach to qualitative data analysis—a deductive approach, essentially testing an existing theory.

Analysing in-depth interviews using a deductive approach

Catherine: I transcribed all my interviews and I had pre-set categories drawn out of the theory. From the theory I drew out what you would call third order concepts, which were theories. First order concepts were just descriptors, which I'd cut up into second order ones—another level of analysis, then into the third order. So I went through all the interviews once, did the first order analysis, then went through them again and looked at the [second order concepts]. I used *The Ethnograph.*

Yvonne: What happened in the first order analysis?

Catherine: I read the interviews through without my schema [of concepts in neo-institutional theory]. Everything that I thought was interesting I coded and gave a code word. It was a purely descriptive process and I ended up with a coding scheme of about 50 or 60 descriptors. I then pulled out each of those descriptors, had a look at them and did searches on them to see what they were saying. They would either split into higher order concepts or sometimes two descriptors would come into one to be a higher order concept. I then went back and re-coded all the interviews and found second order concepts. Sat back, felt sick. Went back to the schema that I'd developed from the theory, extracted all those concepts and printed them out.

Yvonne: These are your second order concepts?

Catherine: The second order ones. And then I looked at them according to the theoretical schema and I re-coded the whole thing again. So after three lots of coding I ended up with conceptual indicators and there were beautiful examples of all of this stuff coming out. It worked, but it was very tiresome . . .

Yvonne: Could you have gone straight to the higher order concepts—used your schema right from the start—or did you need to go through those stages?

Catherine: In hindsight, I reckon I could have. I mean I didn't because I was learning as I went along, but I've noticed since then when I've been doing this sort of thing that I could just pull [the schema] out and go straight to the interviews. But the interesting thing was that I got a research assistant and tried to get her to do the same thing. She couldn't do it, just could not do it. She could do the descriptive stuff but she couldn't do what I was doing, which was going, 'Oh yes, I know that, that's an indicator', but it's just confidence and I think it is two levels of confidence. One is I know the theory so well, and because I've applied it once I know now what it is when I see it. I can see it and I go, 'Oh yes, that's so and so.' So, I can see how researchers get quicker and quicker . . . I'm now a more experienced researcher, more familiar with the theory, and I trust my own instincts whereas I didn't do that the first time around—I thought I was stupid and couldn't possibly be right. I felt very unsure of myself about the qualitative analysis in that field. I still feel a little bit uncomfortable with it but I'm getting surer now.

Caroline Thomas—Adopted children speaking

Here Caroline talks about data analysis and, in particular her use of the *NUD*IST* software program, for her interviews with children about their experiences of adoption.

Dorothy: Can you say a little about the data collection and analysis process? For instance, you did a content analysis and chose to use *NUD*IST*, is that right?

Caroline: We were discouraged from doing it because of the time needed to transcribe, code and then to use the volumes of material that *NUD*IST* sorts and reproduces for you. But I wanted to be sure that I had actually surveyed the breadth of the material and I wanted to try to guard against being too selective on the basis of what had stayed with me . . . Although this was an exploratory study, I still wanted to be able to convey whether the views expressed [by a child] were unusual or whether they were common. I wanted to try to see the patterns, to try to get some sense of the proportions of children who said similar things. I knew that the findings were not statistically significant but I thought it was important to know whether what was being quoted was a one-off example of an extreme case or whether there was some commonality.

Dorothy: Did you look at, say, whether you were getting certain types of responses in relation to the gender of the child or the age at which the child was placed for adoption?

Caroline: We did think about doing that but given that it was such a small sample and that not all the children had been asked the same questions . . . we decided not to in the end.

Dorothy: So in this exploratory study you were interested in the overall themes that are coming through about the adoption process—the chronology of those points of the process you've identified. And were you happy with what *NUD*IST* did for you?

Caroline: Yes. I loved it. I know there are people who don't like using it and who find it cumbersome and time consuming but if I did the exercise again I would want to use a similar tool. I had too elaborate a coding system and consequently the coding of the transcripts took longer than it should have. But given it was the first time I'd used that sort of tool for looking at interview material, it wasn't a surprise that I'd over-catered rather than under-catered with the coding. I would use fewer sub-codes and more global codes, I think, in future.

Comments

At the beginning of this chapter we said we did not intend to provide a comprehensive coverage of qualitative data analysis—the diversity of approaches is far too great and there are many excellent sources for this information. Instead, we provided more general comments about some of the processes common to a range of qualitative data analysis approaches.

These four stories continue that theme. They don't provide a definitive recipe for qualitative data analysis, either individually or in composite. They do provide some glimpses of what happens in practice, how some researchers have gone about their analysis.

They also highlight the crucial role of the researcher who, whatever approach is being used, has to make many decisions about what actually to do in practice.

Qualitative data analysis is a dynamic process and no method can stand in isolation from the world of research practice. Any approach is mediated by the researcher and is only as good as its capacity to assist the researcher to make sense of the data collected. This is not meant to imply an 'anything goes' approach to data analysis. It is always incumbent on the researcher to be rigorous and purposeful, to be clear about the steps taken in data analysis and to be able to defend those steps. This is arguably even more so in qualitative research where there are many possible approaches and where the researcher is so integral an instrument at every stage of the process. The stories presented here, part of the accumulated experience of qualitative researchers, have a part in the continuing evolution of the complex world of qualitative data analysis.

8

Presenting and writing up

Presentation and writing up are integral parts of the research process—no research is completed until it has been reported on. Any one study may be reported in a variety of forms, each with a different purpose and directed at a different audience. It is in fact rare for research findings to be presented in just one form. Where research has been funded, there will be formal reporting requirements. Where research participants have shared their experiences in good faith for the research to be used to create awareness of some issue or problem or to highlight implications for practice or policy, there is an added responsibility to report. Richardson (1990) provides a practical account of the publication of her research on single women involved in long-term relationships with married men in three forms: as a popular book, *The New Other Woman* (1985), an academic journal article (1988) and an article for a mass-circulation magazine (1986).

Presentation and writing up are, of course, just part of the process of ensuring that research findings are directed in such a way that they make a difference to our understanding of particular issues or problems and to how we, as a society, respond to them. Program evaluation writers (Alkin, 1990; Weiss, 1990; Patton, 1997; Owen & Rogers, 1999) commonly draw a distinction between the dissemination of evaluation findings and their use—a distinction that is equally relevant for all social research. Dissemination is a crucial first step but it in no way guarantees use. There are clearly limits to the researcher's control over if and how their research will be used. Political considerations, even fashions in ideas, will influence whether research gets taken up by practitioners or policy-makers. While we tend to think of use as instrumental use, leading to some tangible action, some have argued for a wider definition. Weiss and Bucuvalas introduced the notion of conceptual use, or enlightenment, that could influence thinking about a program without leading to immediate action.

> Research that challenges accepted ideas, arrangements, programs and institutions cannot readily be put to work in a direct and immediate way. It cannot be plugged in to solve problems, particularly when it runs up against the antagonism of interests embodied within the current political balance. But decision-makers' ratings of research indicate that such research can contribute to their work and the work of other appropriate decision-makers. It can *enlighten* them. They do not necessarily apply it *in the short term*, but it affects the way they think about issues and gradually it can affect what they do (Weiss & Bucuvalas, 1980, p. 98).

Owen and Rogers (1999) suggest, in fact, that some form of conceptual use always precedes instrumental use. Cousins and Leithwood (1986) suggest six factors that may influence the utilisation of a particular piece of research: the quality of the research, the credibility of the researcher, the relevance of the research to the needs of decision-makers, the clarity of communication with potential users during and after the research, the nature and implications of the findings, and the timeliness of reporting. We talk more about the impact of research—the shift from research back to practice—in the following chapter.

There are many publications whose purpose is to help researchers, and others, write better. These focus variously on writing style (Murphy, 1985; Strunk & White, 2000), on the process and experience of writing (Woods, 1985; Becker, 1986; Wolcott, 1990; Lofland & Lofland, 1995) and on writing for particular purposes, such as for a thesis (Lewins, 1993; Rountree & Laing, 1996; Anderson & Poole, 1998) or a journal article (Williams & Hopps, 1988; Pirkis & Gardner, 1998).

We do not go over this ground here. Rather, we focus on ways of presenting qualitative findings, including decisions about voice (whose voice/s to present) and decisions about structuring findings. The latter is not an easy task, as data are often voluminous and of their very nature reflect a diversity of experiences and perspectives, defying easy or neat categorisation. This is followed by discussion of some possibilities for alternative modes of presentation.

We also return to Liz Kelly, talking about how she structures qualitative findings; to Tim and Wendy Booth, talking about their approach to writing up the stories of inarticulate research participants; to Cheryl Tilse, talking about presenting findings to different audiences and for different purposes; and to Anne Coleman, talking about the public research readings she held for homeless people.

Whose voices?

One of the most important decisions to make in writing up research is what voices to use—whose stories are they and who is telling them (Wolcott, 1990)? This may well change for different parts of the report. For example, the methodology, the research process and the reasons for conducting the research will, in most cases, be told from the researcher's point of view, whereas other sections may include a combination of researcher and participant voices. There may, of course, be multiple researcher voices, just as there will be multiple participant voices. This will be so where research has been conducted in a team; for participatory and action research, at least some of the voices will be both researcher and participant. It is inevitable that these voices will at times be competing and contradictory—one of the challenges of writing up qualitative research is to find a place for all the perspectives involved.

Padgett (1998) suggests two dimensions that relate to the question of voice—the 'etic-emic' and the 'reflexive-nonreflexive'. The etic-emic dimension relates to the extent to which a report is written from the perspective of the research participants (emic) or of an 'objective' outsider (etic). The nonreflexive-reflexive dimension reflects the extent to which the researcher's experiences and perspectives are included in the report. By intersecting the dimensions, we can imagine four quadrants, each representing a different approach to writing a report.

The etic-nonreflexive report approximates the classic 'realist tale' (van Maanen, 1988), written in the third person, emphasising the researcher's authority to report the lives of others, but containing little of the researcher themselves. The emic-nonreflexive report, characterised by ethnomethodological and phenomenological approaches, emphasises the lived experience of research participants, with limited interpretation by the researcher (Holstein & Gubrium, 1994). Etic-reflexive reports reflect a combination approach in that they present a largely etic report of research findings but include additional sections detailing the researcher's experiences of the research—how their presence may have impacted on the research and how the research impacted on them. This approach serves two functions. It reports the substantive content of the research but also takes seriously issues of reactivity and reflexivity. It is commonly used for formal presentations such as a thesis. Emic-reflexive reports are 'confessional tales' (van Maanen, 1988) that focus largely on the researcher's perspectives. They contribute to our understanding of how research really happens (Hyde, 1994; Moran-Ellis, 1996) but they do not substitute for a research report.

We recommend an approach that keeps the researcher in but does not so privilege the researcher's experiences that participants' voices are lost or overshadowed. The researcher is, however, central to any qualitative research and this should be reflected in the written report. At the least this should include material on how the research came to be conducted and any assumptions the researcher brings to the work—their positioning in relation to participants, to the broader topic, their professional background, and so on. It also makes sense to include the researcher's active voice in the methodology and findings. How the research is conducted, how the analysis unfolds, what patterns the researcher identifies, what theoretical sense they make of it and the approach to writing up are all researcher-dependent choices and should be acknowledged as such.

Direct quotations from participants are integral to qualitative research reports—they bring the research to life. They also show the reader the evidence upon which the researcher's interpretations are based. But overuse of quotes can become tedious and the point being made can get lost in the words. Wolcott's advice is to the point: 'Save the best and drop the rest' (1990, p. 67). He also cautions against being overly wedded to reporting examples of subtle differences in the data that are unlikely to be recognised by readers who are not as immersed in the study as the researcher is. 'Most of us see and hear our informants as we enter their words onto a manuscript. We forget that our readers cannot do that; for them, the words remain lifeless on the page, and the repetition of materials that are virtually identical becomes tedious' (1990, p. 68).

In studies where participants may be readily identifiable, either to themselves or to others, confidentiality requires that what individuals actually said be disguised. In such cases it may be wiser to rely on aggregate comments at a higher level of generality than to make liberal use of direct quotes.

Structuring qualitative findings

Inevitably, decisions have to be made about how to order the data in the written report. Where the research has focused on a social setting, say a child protection office, it may lend itself to being reported according to particular aspects of the setting (worker–client interviews, court work, staff meetings or informal staff interactions), different stages of assessment and intervention, or the perspectives of different participants (parents, children, child protection workers, managers, or professionals from other agencies).

Where there are several equally plausible and effective ways of structuring the report, the purpose and overall framing of the study will help in making the choice. If a study was, for example, about emotional experiences in marriage, the report may lend itself to being structured according to a range of emotions. If the study was a comparison of emotional experiences across a range of relationships, then the report may be equally well structured according to emotions or to different types of relationships.

Ultimately, the decision rests with the researcher as to which structure is going to provide the most effective vehicle for the findings. What is the message and how can it best be got across? Remember, though, the simpler the better—the structure should never become so complex or cluttered that it gets in the way of the content. Yvonne Darlington structured her study of women who had been sexually abused as children (1996) into three broad topic areas: impact on self, impact on relationships with others and experiences of professional intervention, healing and recovery. This provided a manageable structure for reporting a huge array of data.

Becker's position is that there is no 'one right way' to organise written research reports. He understood that his thesis on schoolteachers' evaluations of their relationships with students, parents, the principal and other teachers could be organised around kinds of schools or kinds of work relations.

> Whichever way I chose, I would have to describe teachers and
> working-class kids, teachers and slum school colleagues, teachers and

the principals of middle-class schools, and all the other combinations of relations and school types created by cross-classifying relation and class . . . Either way, I would report the same results (although in a different order) and arrive at essentially the same conclusions (though the terms they were put in and their emphases would differ). What I said about the implications for social science theory and social policy would differ, naturally. If I used my results to answer different questions, the answers would look different. But none of that would affect the work that lay immediately ahead of me as I began writing my thesis. Why worry about it? (Becker, 1986, p. 58).

While quantitative studies lend themselves more naturally to the succinct presentation of results and discussion of relevant findings, the distinction can be less clear-cut in qualitative research, where description and interpretation are more closely interwoven. We have found it helpful to divide a report into major topic areas and to include a separate discussion section within each, after the thematic description. In this way, the author's interpretation does not become too intermingled with the voices of the research participants, but occurs close enough to the thematic analysis to allow the reader to see how it has been interpreted. Whatever choice is made, it is important to be clear about who is talking at any point.

We have been talking particularly about qualitative studies that focus closely on participants' accounts and draw their interpretations from the data, developing theory using an inductive logic. These comments are less applicable to theory testing studies. The latter tend to be more conceptually driven than data driven and the kinds of writing-up issues we have been addressing often do not arise—the theory being tested, or the conceptual framework driving the study, also provides the structure for the report.

In writing up qualitative research it is not always immediately obvious what tense should be used for the various parts of the report. This is especially so in studies which include direct quotes from participants, where the primary inclination will often be to present them in as immediate a way as possible. Wolcott provides useful advice, however, in the suggestion to write descriptive passages in the past tense right from the start, even if this seems odd or even disrespectful to participants you may still be working with or whose reported experiences are still vividly in your mind— certainly one works with their words for a long time through the analysis and writing up processes. He says:

By the time your manuscript has gone through many iterations, editorial review, and publication you will discover that the past tense no longer seems so strange, and you will not have left informants forever doing and saying whatever they happened to be doing and saying during your brief tenure (Wolcott, 1990, p. 47).

Is there a book in it?

A question asked by many researchers, especially postgraduate students, is whether they should attempt to publish their research as a book. There are no clear-cut answers. It depends on the nature of the work and whether there is a publisher which considers there is a market for it. Some research reports (theses) form an interlinked whole and it 'makes sense' to keep the bits together—equally, it may not make sense to separate the bits, as the integrity of the work or its potential impact would be diminished. Publishers will primarily be concerned with whether the book will sell, so it needs to be on a topic with reasonably broad and current appeal, and with an identifiable audience.

It is important to get advice. Supervisors and thesis examiners are useful people to start with—they will have read the thesis and may be able to comment on whether they can picture it making the transition from thesis to book. Thesis examiners are often asked to comment on how publishable a work is, and may include specific comments about possible forms of publication in their report.

If you do decide to try to publish a book from the thesis, the first step is to find a publisher. Choosing carefully can save a lot of time. Select as prospective publishers those who are known to include works of the type you want to write in their list and then prepare a book proposal. Any proposal should include the rationale behind the book, a brief outline of each chapter, the proposed word length and the target readership. The book proposal is more than just sharing information about what you would like to do. Its aim is also to convince the publisher that this is a project worth taking on. If you are successful first time, congratulations. If not, consider trying again. There are many reasons why a publisher won't accept a project at a particular time; some may suggest other publishers you could approach.

Writing a book from a thesis is always a major task that requires hard decisions about what is left in and what goes out. That can be difficult at first, after all the time spent working on the great labour of love that is a thesis. It is probably a good idea to leave it a while anyway—to get some distance from it. Consider writing some journal articles in the meantime—this is often easier, as they tend to be chunks that can be pulled out without disturbing 'the thesis' itself.

In writing a book based on a thesis, you may find that some prominent sections of the thesis take up only a small part of the book and new sections may have to be written. The literature will always need to be updated. While it is difficult to generalise, the book will tend to be shorter overall, the literature review will be less exhaustive, and the methodology will occupy a less prominent position. Depending on the audience, the methodology may best be included as an appendix. As a general rule, the more scholarly the intended audience the more extensive the methodology will need to be.

Yvonne Darlington rewrote her PhD thesis on women's experiences of childhood sexual abuse (1993) as a book for a practitioner audience (1996). This required considerable restructuring of the original material: the book is less than half the size of the thesis; the methodology is placed as an appendix, and greatly summarised; the literature review is shorter and more targeted to the central content of the book; and one major section of findings—the women's remembered experiences of abuse and its impact in childhood—does not appear, as the book is focused on longer-term impact, experiences of counselling and processes of healing and recovery.

Alternative forms of presentation

Research need not be disseminated only in written form. Paget had excerpts of her research on mis-communications between doctor and patient adapted and presented as a piece of formal theatre, staged and performed by theatre students. The performance text was drawn from a written report on the research, including the doctor–patient exchanges as well as Paget's analysis. Paget says of this work:

> Performance promises a far richer and more subtle science of culture than the analytic text can establish. But it makes different demands. It requires a narrative, drama, action, and a point of view. This work succeeded as theater because the original text had a narrator who

reported dramatic events, because it contained a real dialogue, and, also, because it had a good reason to be told (Paget, 1990, p. 152).

In a different but equally innovative approach, Becker, McCall and Morris (1989; see also McCall, Becker & Meshejian, 1990) have conducted staged readings of their research on the social organisation of professional theatre. In these theatrical presentations, the researchers are the performers, talking as themselves but also taking on the roles of research participants. Theirs presents an innovative approach/response to 'telling it like it is'. First, there is room for all three researchers' voices in the presentation of the research: 'To reduce our three voices to the single authorial voice in a conventional social science text (and thus hide our negotiations, disagreements, and the ideas we share) would misrepresent the way we produce performance science scripts' (Becker et al., 1989, p. 94). They also argue that the research participants' voices come through more strongly in the performance medium:

> We let the voices of the people who talked to us be heard more fully than usual, with less intervention by us, in long speeches or in conversations, not in short quotes used as evidence for the generalizations we want to make. Long quotes contain more 'noise', more material that isn't exactly about the point being made. You can't disguise the speaker's own meaning when you use long quotes. You can't make them say just what you want the audience to hear and no more (1989, p. 95).

Both have the effect of deprivileging the researcher:

> Turning the sociologists into characters in the script makes them less authoritative and easier to argue with, especially if you give them several voices and let them disagree with each other. Scripts are 'multivocal'—this one has twenty-five voices speaking—and the multivocality further deprivileges the analyst (1989, p. 95).

In Caroline Thomas and her colleagues' study on older adopted children (Thomas et al., 1999), the researchers used an interesting way to protect the confidentiality of the children while allowing what they had to say to be heard verbatim in the public domain. They taperecorded other children reading the transcripts of the adopted children's interviews, playing the recordings to prospective adoptive parents and social workers during their training sessions to enable them to appreciate the subjective experiences of adopted children in their own words. This protected the privacy of the adopted children while evocatively conveying their experiences much more powerfully than the written word would have allowed.

Stories from the field

This chapter's stories are again drawn from our interviews with researchers. Readers who are interested in the published work of these researchers and the other researchers interviewed for this book can follow-up the references in the bibliography.

Liz Kelly—Domestic violence matters

Here Liz talks about her preferred approach to writing up mixed methods research. Her position that qualitative and quantitative methods are equal but different—each making a unique contribution to any study—is reflected in her resolve to integrate the findings from both approaches in written reports on her research (Kelly, 1999).

Writing up a mixed methods study

Yvonne: How do you write up a mixed methods study?

Liz: I think with enormous difficulty. Looking at *Domestic Violence Matters* now, I don't think I entirely succeeded. The chapter on crisis intervention I really like, I think it works. It draws on different parts of the data and there is a thread weaving through it that different parts of the data illuminate and help explore. I think the chapter on the police is clumsy and dense and tries to use too much of the data without distilling it. That was the hardest one to do partly because the data was incomplete. The information that we ought to have had from the police wasn't available, so it was having to kind of wander around, without having a central core . . .

I think the thing for me is that if you have a clear thread or couple of threads that you can follow and the data weaves into this thread, then it is okay, then you can work out which data are 'setting-the-scene' and come at the beginning, which are the more complex data in the middle and then which are the data that give you some kind of clear insights. If you don't have that, or there are too many possible threads to follow, then it is actually quite difficult, because it's hard to know what to select . . . whether this bit of data goes with this, or with that. I suppose one of the things you do, is that you use the more quantitative data as the scene-setting—this is how many, this is how much of this, how much of that—and then the qualitative data enables you to explore. I think a lot of times qualitative data are used as a kind of illustration, a sort of more accessible description, but there are also other ways that you use it. One of the ways we use it is to show contradiction. For example, there is one lot of police officers who understand arrest in this way, and another lot of police officers who understand arrest in a different way. Qualitative data helps us to communicate some of the complexity and the dilemmas as well. Quantitative data can't give you a sense of the actual messiness of real life, and qualitative data can show you that—okay, yes, there are some police officers who are offensive and whatever, and there are some who are great, but most of them are struggling to know what to do, and to make sense of often conflicting messages. I don't think I was as clear about that when I wrote it, as I am now, and I don't think that it is stated there as strongly as I would now.

Yvonne: Was that about having time and distance from the study, or something else?

Liz: It is partly that this was the first piece of research where the police were subjects, and it is partly through talking with researchers from other countries who have also done research on the police, in relation to domestic violence. In dialogue, I think I have come to see that actually, unintentionally, the demands of the women's movement have placed the police in a quite complicated position, because on the one hand the demand has been for more victim-centred and empathetic understandings in response, but on the other hand to respond to domestic violence as a crime . . . and I think *Domestic Violence Matters* was part of a journey where I arrived at this understanding, but when I was writing it up I hadn't quite grasped it with the clarity I have now. Had I [had that clarity], I think that would have been the thread in the police chapter that would have given it a different feel, and would have enabled me to move in and out of the qualitative and quantitative in a way that had a sense of direction. I feel that chapter provides lots and lots of information, and not enough signposts as to why is this information here, what is it doing . . .

Yvonne: So what you do in practice is to interweave the qualitative and quantitative data, in the same chapter, in the same section even . . .

Liz: And the interpretative, conceptual, analytic, all those things that are what the researcher's job is in relation to this material, to find the thread . . . I don't think I would know how to write it in any other way now, which is interesting and it hasn't been a principled decision to do this with some kind of deeply sophisticated rationale at all. I think it is to do with how I understand multi-methods, but these things you do on a subconscious level without [realising]—you are making me bring to the surface things that are just implicit in my work—that I do see the two kinds of data as being in a dialogue with each other. Sometimes they just illuminate each other, and sometimes it is about saying it is all very well to have these numbers, but actually sitting underneath these numbers is a much more complex, difficult and dilemma-filled reality. The numbers don't enable you to know that, but you need to know it if you are going to do anything useful, or if you are going to even understand it properly. So to me they need to be together to illuminate, either in a sort of confirmational way, or in a way that it is more complicated than that.

Yvonne: Do you see the methods as more or less equal, or at the end of the day does one become more influential than the other? Or does that depend on the context of where you are reporting?

Liz: Well, there is my perception and [there are] external perceptions. I see them as equivalent and as necessary to one another. They are part of the process of discovery and sense-making of the material, but I know that for policy-makers it is numbers that count, while for practitioners it is often the experiential that counts. So again, you know if you are trying to do this difficult job of writing for multiple audiences then I think that is a reason for trying to use them together, because you are trying to speak to the audiences in the way that they find easiest to absorb or accept, or be influenced by, information. One of our guiding principles is to create knowledge that is of use to those who are in the position to make a difference, and there are lots of audiences that are in a position to make a difference, different kinds of differences. So our ambition is always to try to speak to audiences simultaneously.

Cheryl Tilse—The long goodbye

Cheryl has presented her work, in verbal and written form, to several different audiences and in a range of formats (Tilse, 1996, 1997a, 1997b). Here she talks about how she has tailored the content and process of presentation for different audiences.

Presenting research to different audiences

Cheryl: Some of the things were the same. I always thought that the strength was in the stories and the quotes— I think they're very compelling and they're still with me. Some of these I wrote back in 1994, but the stories are still there and the quotes are still there so I think I let a lot of it speak for itself. But I do put an interpretation on it. With the participants [relatives of nursing home residents] I was really keen for them to see themselves in it. So I wrote lots of quotes and then said, 'But other people said similar things to you', and all of that. For the practitioners [nursing home staff] I was really keen not to have a critique of what they did but to say 'here's a way of understanding what some

170

of the things that bother you are about—why families
are so demanding and why older men don't seem to
know what to do when they come and what can you
do about it'. So I was trying to get some practice ideas
and some new thinking. So it was very much—I didn't
talk about roles, resources, rights and relationships—
at a human level, and always through examples,
always grounded in trying to convince them I knew
what I was talking about because I'd talked to older
people and this is what I had seen happen. Although
it's all about human relationships and meaning, I've
always seen it as a policy thesis, about understanding
a key policy issue of residential care of older people
and trying to make policy more receptive to a broader
approach to understanding what some things are
about. It's about how you incorporate meaning to
activities such as family participation rather than
simply rational decision-making models. So I write
very differently for the policy audience. At a policy
conference you talk in terms of policy and use the
same examples to question the policy, I suppose. So
the examples are the same, it's just what you select
and what you leave out and the way you write that are
different. But it's more similar than you would imagine
at times because it's the same stories, [just] told with
a different level in mind. For practice audiences I was
saying that these are the sorts of things people told me
about, this is what happened for them and this is how
I saw some people respond to it and it seemed to work
well. So I think that's the strength of the qualitative
material, that it really speaks for itself a lot. You
can just frame it. All your writing is targeted at an
audience—you know who you're talking to and the
points you want to make, but the qualitative data is so
rich it speaks for itself . . . and it is very powerful.

Tim and Wendy Booth—Parenting under pressure

Here Tim talks about the challenges involved in writing up—and
doing justice to—the accounts of people with an intellectual

disability. He draws on their study of parents with a learning difficulty (Booth & Booth, 1994a) as well as that of children of parents with a learning difficulty (Booth & Booth, 1996).

An approach to writing up the stories of inarticulate informants

Tim: The challenge is how do you tell the story? How do you tell the stories of people who lack words? . . . In the case of the group of people that we are talking about, the inherent incoherence of most transcripts may be exaggerated because they lack the same command of grammar, the same vocabulary and the same oratorical skills. Now, if as a researcher you believe in the notion of being absolutely true to the data that you collect, and only presenting the material verbatim, frankly, most of the time you would end up with an incoherent story. You wouldn't be able to use it to convey information to a reader, because the reader wouldn't be able to penetrate the prose, lacking the kind of struts and supports that the interviewer or researcher had—prior knowledge of the person, an understanding of their lives, experience of the way in which they express themselves. Lacking all that and asking a reader to make sense of a transcript is presenting them with an impossible task and actually is also doing a disservice to the informant, because it emphasises their [inarticulateness], when, in context, they might very well have been able to express themselves . . . So there is a real challenge there for researchers, in the sense of how do you cope with this quite fundamental dilemma . . . My considered view, based upon ten years of research, is that while people have the stories, and we have the words, we can lend them the words to enable them to tell their stories. That in itself brings all kinds of ethical issues, issues of legitimation and representation, which I would gladly expand on at length, but I am sure you are not here to listen to me go on about it now, though it is a real challenge.

Yvonne: How do you deal with some of those issues? You are saying if you don't in a sense take over and write the story, it is not going to get told, but what kind of safe-guards do you build in?

Tim: I suppose in thinking about how you do it, I would probably hold in my mind a chapter that appeared in the growing up with parents who have learning diffi-culties book [Booth & Booth, 1996], which takes the form of a conversation between two sisters. Many of the techniques that we used in constructing that chapter are techniques that would apply to our work generally. Everything that is in the chapter was spoken by the informants—nothing has been added, but the order of the words isn't necessarily the same. The ordering of the sentences isn't necessarily the same. There have been cuts made, elisions, and the material has been very heavily edited into a coherent text that is true to their story and was validated by the inform-ants, in that they were presented with the text, and they okayed it.

Anne Coleman—Five star motels

As part of the process of feeding back findings to the people who had participated in her study (Coleman, 2001), Anne conducted a series of research readings of her work. While she did not talk of her presentation of findings as performance, Anne's oral presentation of her work to the homeless people in her study has some parallels with performance science, albeit in a less formal way.

Research readings for homeless people

Anne: This was not entirely satisfactory, but it was the best I could do—I wanted to take the whole of the thesis back to people and say 'Is it all put together okay?' Now obviously I knew that a large number of people wouldn't give a damn about the literature review or what I said in the methodology, so I did some readings at a drop-in centre [that] I knew a lot of these people accessed. Again I flagged them with the graphic image and I went down there and read big sections of it to some people . . .

Yvonne: What happened at the readings? What would a typical one have been like?

Anne: This one is typical at one extreme. There was just one guy and we spent about three hours together. That was really productive because he was interested not just in the findings and hearing the bits about him but he was interested in all of it. So I actually got to read some of the methodology and talk about some of those issues with him. That was just delightful. And then another typical one was when quite a few Murris turned up one day and there were quite a few other people. It was payday, and the atmosphere was, 'We've all had some drinks, we're just going to go up to the club and Anne's going to tell us a story.' And that was totally different. It was shorter. It was probably only maybe an hour and a half because of course people had other things to do and they wanted to go and have another drink. That particular session was about acknowledgement for them—I'd start reading and they'd say, 'No, no, no, read that other bit. Read us another bit about somebody saying something. Tell us a bit more about that.'

Yvonne: So they wanted the bits where they were quoted?

Anne: Yes. 'Where are we? Where are we in there? Yeah, we know what you think Anne. That's fascinating but we've heard it all before.' So that was really like just selected bits but it was a good process of confirmation for me at the end . . . at every session, the consistent thing was that for the first half an hour it was like I was the expert. Nobody would say anything, they'd just sit there. And once they'd warmed up they'd start to ask you questions or they'd start to say things, but when it got to the 'read us our bits' stage, I'd always get that confirmation. You'd see people, even the people who said nothing, smiling or nodding, as if to say 'Oh yeah, I know that one. Oh yeah, she got that right. Oh yes, we know what that feels like.' So I guess that's not the way that people usually get their [research] verified but with that group of people that was a strong verification.

Anne felt pleased with the readings and believes this approach to presenting findings has implications beyond her study:

> *Anne:* I think that this has overcome one of those big methodological gaps in research with people in this area about how do you do feed back. They've got really good communication networks so as long as you keep tapped into the network you can get the information out about what you're going to do. And I now think that it's a good way. Some people said, 'We couldn't care less.' Others, 'Look, we know you, we know what you're going to say. It's all right with us. We trust you', but other people were really keen. They wanted to hear it.

Comments

These four stories illustrate a variety of approaches to presenting qualitative research to diverse audiences. They all retain the richness and uniqueness of the data, whether in Liz Kelly's attempt to integrate and communicate both the numbers and the underlying messiness, Cheryl Tilse's use of quotations from spouses to illuminate a policy point, or Anne Coleman's reading back to homeless people what they had said during the research. The researchers are aware of the power of qualitative research to move audiences, but they do this always with a particular purpose and audience in mind. People's stories are treated respectfully and not used for gratuitous effect. Tim Booth is also aware of the communicative potential of the stories of his participants with learning difficulties but faced the dilemma that this would largely be lost if he used just their verbatim accounts. He opted instead to edit the text to make the story more easily accessible to the audience.

These excerpts also illustrate that writing up and dissemination are processes that need not end there. The purpose of research in the human services is always to have some impact, for some change to occur as a result of the work—whether a direct instrumental effect in the form of changes to practice or policy or a more general contribution to the development of thinking in an area. We focus on the impact of research in the final chapter. There is not necessarily a marked delineation between these stages. While research dissemination starts in earnest at the completion of a project, it also happens along the way—research can have an impact at any stage.

9

Epilogue: From research to practice, programs and politics

We began this journey looking at how qualitative research can be generated from the swampy lowland of practice in the human services. We end it by examining the impact of such research, thus completing the loop back to practice. It is not always easy to identify the impact of research. Some studies have an obvious and immediate effect while the effects of others may be almost imperceptible, particularly in the short term. It is also hard to differentiate the impact of one study from that of others as one piece of research can lead to another, creating multiple ripples in a reservoir of research and practice in which it is impossible to determine the ripple from a particular stone.

The researcher may not be aware of the impact which a study has, just as human services managers, policy-makers and practitioners may not be fully aware of the research which is influencing them in their decisions. In this chapter we look briefly at how qualitative research in the human services can be used to enhance the response of the service system and the broader community to complex human problems. We conclude by giving a few examples from our interviews with researchers.

While it will mostly be people other than researchers who will put into practice the implications of their findings, researchers have an important role to play in determining the impact of their study. Making recommendations in the most effective ways possible is a key part of this. Surprisingly, very little attention has been given in the research literature on how to do this. Patton, an expert in qualitative program evaluation, commented that:

> Recommendations have long troubled me because they have seemed the weakest part of evaluation. We have made enormous progress in ways of studying programs, methodological diversity, and a variety of data-collection techniques and designs. The pay off from these advances comes in the recommendations we make. But we have made very little progress in how to construct useful recommendations (Patton, 1988, p. 90).

Perhaps there needs to be a research project on how best to write research recommendations! Below is a summary of the suggestions which Hendricks and Papagiannis (1990, pp. 122–5) have proposed for making recommendations in relation to program evaluation. They are applicable also to other types of research.

- Consider all issues in your evaluation to be 'fair game' for recommendations, not just those the research was designed to investigate.
- Don't wait until the end of your evaluation to begin thinking about recommendations—record possible recommendations from the commencement of data collection.
- Draw possible recommendations from a wide variety of sources, including earlier studies of similar programs and program staff of different levels in the organisation.
- Work closely with agency personnel throughout the process to minimise the threat which unexpected recommendations can pose, and engage stakeholders who have the power to implement them.
- Consider the contexts into which the recommendations must fit and make realistic recommendations, thinking carefully before recommending fundamental changes.
- Decide how specific you want your recommendations to be and consider the possibility of providing options for decision-makers.
- Show the future implications of your recommendations in as much detail as possible and consider planning an implementation strategy and, if invited, consider becoming involved in the implementation itself.
- Make your recommendations easy for decision-makers to understand, categorising them in meaningful ways (for example, short-term and long-term) and adapt the way recommendations

are presented to the way in which the decision-makers normally receive information.

The suggestions above are focused on making recommendations in relation to the research site of a particular program which has been evaluated. Most research will have implications which go well beyond a specific research site, and may need to be disseminated in different ways to different audiences, as was discussed in the previous chapter. The external environment will also greatly influence whether there is a receptive climate for the research. Often the origin of the research occurs within a particular policy and social context which also affects how it is received. However, given the dynamic and turbulent field of the human services, the research may be finally delivered in a very different context to that in which it was conceived. This may mean that the findings are seen as dated and so are easily passed over.

Conversely, the findings can sometimes take on greater salience in an external environment which has changed significantly since the research commenced. An example of this is the study on adoption experiences of older children undertaken by Caroline Thomas and her colleagues. The publication of the book coincided with very high-level political attention on the issue of children languishing in institutions when they were eligible for adoption. This helped to give the study a higher profile than it might otherwise have received.

When making recommendations researchers need to be mindful of the context of their study in terms of its time and place. Extrapolating the findings of a study to other contexts is always a central issue in human services. Researchers and those who utilise research must therefore be very aware of the core components of the context in which the research was done and the core components of the context in which the recommendations arising from it may be implemented.

Sometimes the most important contextual components of both the research site and where it is hoped to apply the findings are not very visible, as they tend to be taken for granted. This is a particular challenge when crossing different service systems in the human services field, as very different legislation and service systems exist across regions and states, as do demographic differences. The challenge is even greater when crossing national and cultural boundaries.

In industry this process is called 'technology transfer' but in relation to the human services the term does not give sufficient salience to the contextual features which need to be considered. We prefer to describe it as a process of transplanting innovation across different landscapes. The metaphor of taking a plant from the climatic and soil conditions in which it originally grew and trying to grow it elsewhere draws awareness to the different contextual characteristics which must be considered if the transplant is to be successful. The researcher will need to think carefully about what needs to be changed to make the program or policy fit the context into which it is being introduced, while being mindful of the risk of damaging what might be the core ingredients which make a program work.

There is obviously a trade-off between maintaining the integrity of a model and adapting it to fit new contexts. In Dorothy Scott's child protection assessment study (outlined in Chapter 2), the conflict between various organisations in the child protection system was particularly intense during the period of data collection. This was precisely why the study investigated inter-organisational and inter-professional conflict—but by the time the research was completed, the highly politicised controversies surrounding the child protection system had diminished. The question then arose as to how applicable the findings and recommendations were in relation to the new context.

Thus the generalisability and transferability of research are in direct proportion to the degree to which the findings are context-bound. This is true for both quantitative and qualitative research. In making recommendations researchers need to acknowledge the possible limitations on the transferability of their studies, while not minimising the significance of the study's findings to other settings.

The researcher's role may go beyond dissemination and making recommendations. Some human services researchers are actively involved in a strategic process of developmental research which Fraser and Leavitt (1990) have described as 'mission-oriented research and entrepreneurship'. In developmental research of this nature the evaluation is just one part of the process described by Thomas (1978) as consisting of the following phases:

- Analysis (identification of need)
- Development (designing the social technology)
- Evaluation (assessing the program)

- Diffusion (disseminating information)
- Adoption (implementing the program).

Fraser and Leavitt (1990) use the US model of intensive family-based services, 'Homebuilders', as a case study of this type of research, which typically involves a large number of people and organisations. However, most research in the human services will not be part of such a linear strategic process, as some of the following stories illustrate well.

Stories from the field

We have selected quite a few of our stories to highlight the impact that qualitative research in the human services can have, both in the short term, sometimes commencing during the study itself, through to the long term. The first one we present is Anne Coleman's study (2001), which was still in progress at the time we interviewed her. We were interested in finding out about the impact that research may have, even at such an early stage. This is followed with an excerpt from the interview with Cheryl Tilse. It picks up from the previous chapter and relates to reaching audiences beyond the research sites through conference presentations and media interviews (Tilse, 1996). Caroline Thomas then speaks briefly about the impact her adoption study has had in the year since its publication (Thomas, 1999), and how the political environment in which it was released gave it a special salience. Liz Kelly discusses how her study's different conceptualisation of domestic violence intervention struck a chord with workers in the field of family violence (Kelly, 1999). Jackie Sanders also talks about how the research she has done with Robyn Munford has been used by a range of people, from students and practitioners to policy-makers and funding sources. We conclude with Dorothy Scott reflecting on the long-term outcomes of her research undertaken with maternal and child health nurses in the early 1980s (Scott, 1987a, 1987b, 1992).

Anne Coleman—Five star motels

Anne: Yes, I've quite a strong sense of [impact] now . . . I've talked to a lot of people in the last ten years, in the

bureaucracy, in homelessness services and in politics
. . . and the sorts of things I've said are simply that it's
pointless to move people on. These are the spaces that
capitalism has left for them. If you're now going to tell
them to leave these spaces, where will they go? And
how do you expect that sort of response to be effective? But in the last twelve months, I now hear the
local Councillor saying things like, 'We will no longer
move homeless people on from this area.' Some
people in Brisbane City Council—not necessarily the
top levels—are starting to take on this idea of 'Yes,
that's actually right. These are all the same people
we've been moving on from these spaces for ten years
and they're still the same people so obviously this is
not a very good way to go about it.' So I know that in
terms of the federal government response it's pretty
much unchanged, and I know that the long-term
homeless people whom I've looked at in this research
probably won't be much better off, but I can see a shift
at the local level; in terms of making life different for
the people that I'm concerned about, where it will
make a difference is at the local level. So . . . I feel like
it's been a very useful piece of work already.

Cheryl Tilse—The long goodbye

Cheryl: I didn't change the world. I think I had an impact on all
of the facilities that I worked in, and I certainly spent the
year after I'd written the thesis talking about the need to
understand the perspectives of older spouses. I did a lot
of that—I got invited to the annual general meeting of
the Gerontology Association; I did a talk with staff at a
hospital; and I did a talk for nurses in aged care facilities. So I targeted workers and . . . really I was saying
these older spouses need a voice. I was trying to
increase the understanding of the issues for them. I was
trying to get to front-line workers rather than social
workers or policy workers. I did some in-service training
sessions for some church-run nursing homes where
they brought in all their workers . . . I wrote a report in

practical and simple language that I sent back to the facilities—how to understand the issue, what was it about and what not to do. I know some people read it. I know that that's probably the least likely way of getting information to front-line staff but it's a good way to get it to management.

I know when I talk about [the study] that I can talk in ways that move people. And whenever I present stuff, I always get practitioners saying, 'What can we do? I work in a hospital. How can we address this thing?' I've targeted particular groups in the dementia area—hospitals, social workers—saying you really have to take care of the people who are placing someone with dementia because it's a very traumatic thing and here are the ways you can help and this is what the issues sometimes are . . . I got a call last year, from a social worker in a hospital . . . saying, 'We heard you at the conference and we want to develop a support program for families.' Social workers rang from interstate and talked to me about what they could do; they were working in nursing homes and might be able to set up a program . . . so I talked about a lot of things that you could do in practice and how I'd seen a support group work and what were the elements of one that worked for families.

Geraldine Doogue talked about the study on ABC National Radio and there were articles in the *Sydney Morning Herald* and in the *General Practice* magazine, which meant that it went out to a wider audience. I had phone calls from that, including a GP ringing from another state saying, 'I've got an old man here who's putting his wife in a nursing home. What can I do to help?' . . . I feel that I should have done more with it but it was always a matter of time.

Caroline Thomas—Adopted children speaking

Caroline: The feedback that I've been given has been very positive in terms of its impact, particularly on social work practice. At conferences people tell me it has changed the way they do things, and [that] it's quoted all over the place. Certainly my project director— well, one of them in particular, who has been doing policy-related research for many years—has told me he's pretty sure that it's having more impact than many other studies he's been involved in. I wonder if this is because of its simplicity, in a way . . .

Dorothy: What do you think practitioners will do with it? What would you hope that many practitioners would have learned, fundamentally, about how to work with children in the process of adoption?

Caroline: Because we were fortunate enough to include some of the tools in the book, I hope it will give them inspiration, and some confidence. Perhaps what I didn't manage to convey in the book was how I felt we learned a lot from very good practitioners, who do direct work with children, in our consultation process when we were developing the tools . . . Our whole approach was really about bringing together expertise and views from lots of different sources, including social work practice itself. When I make presentations to practitioners I always feel a little bit uneasy handing back to them what they have given to me. Sometimes I say, depending on the audience, 'Really, you taught me this.'

Liz Kelly—Domestic violence matters

Liz: Interestingly, I think that the study—in terms of the document itself—has been less influential than other things we have done, that we have been paid less money for . . . I think that is partly to do with [the fact] that it stayed in the Home Office for three years after it was finished, which meant that there was a timing issue. Had it come out a year after it was finished when people were asking questions about it—and there was an interest in the outcomes—I think it probably would have had more impact. It has, though, affected how we present material about domestic violence, the things we emphasise in talks, the basic messages . . . too much of the intervention focuses on leaving and the assumption that this is the option you offer women and if they don't want it, then that's their problem, so it has very much shifted our questions and challenges to those who work in the field—there is a whole process before women are ready or able to leave, and too little of the intervention focuses on that. It has also been a challenge to the women's services, who have traditionally provided refuge, which is again about leaving, and we have just written a review for the Home Office . . . about advocacy and outreach approaches and this study has informed that. And I have had feedback from practitioners that the bit that they found the most useful is part of the process analysis where . . . we conceptualise domestic violence in terms of forms of power, positions of power. So there's a part at the end that talks about institutional power, formal power, personal power and gender power and people have said that they find that really helpful in making sense of processes in projects and interagency groups.

Robyn Munford and Jackie Sanders—Working successfully with families

Jackie: I think that [our] research has been one of a number of contributions to the growing interest at a policy level in strengths-based work with families. I know that the research findings have been used in negotiations with funders of family services to help explain why certain funding approaches won't work in practice and to argue for increased recognition in funding contracts for a 'whole person' or 'whole family' approach to funding. We have had lots of positive feedback from practitioners relating to the findings and the endorsement it gives to models of good practice. The materials are used in teaching both practice and research in universities and other tertiary institutions, both [in New Zealand] and in Australia,

185

and we understand that there is interest in them in the United Kingdom as well.

As researchers, we really want to make a contribution to family change—we can't do that directly but we can do it by providing good information to practitioners, managers and policy-makers. From the outset we wanted to produce research that made sense to these people and that they could use, and this has driven our work and continues to drive it. We have always been aware that it is not enough just to do the research and hope that people will find it, so we are very active in circulating our materials and trying hard to make them accessible in as wide a range of settings as we possibly can. We have found people incredibly receptive to our work and that is really pleasing. We try to establish and maintain a dialogue with a wide range of users of our work to keep on hearing what it is they need in terms of information and how they need it delivered to them and then to incorporate that into the work we do.

Dorothy Scott—Identification of post-partum depression

Dorothy: In Chapter 1 I described how my research in the early 1980s with Victorian maternal and child health nurses grew out of my clinical work with women with post-partum psychiatric disorders. My initial goal of increasing the capacity of the maternal and child health service to identify and refer women to psychiatric services was broadened to explore the conditions under which the nurses might encompass maternal emotional and social well-being in their role. I would never have guessed that fifteen years later I would find myself on the steps of the Victorian Parliament with a megaphone in my hand, addressing a large crowd, mostly women pushing prams, demonstrating against government moves to restrict access to the maternal and child health service! In all of the intervening fifteen years, it never felt like I was taking the research down a predetermined pathway—rather

[it] was dragging me along unfamiliar pathways. This was because the time was ripe for the sort of study I ended up doing. Leading maternal and child health nurses were becoming concerned about post-natal depression and keen to broaden their role to encompass maternal emotional and social well-being. The shift in nursing education from a hospital-based apprenticeship model to a university-based professional education some years earlier had helped to create a new generational cohort of nurse practitioners who were more psychologically oriented and who were eager to work in different ways. The study described and conceptualised the clinical judgement of exemplary maternal and child health nurses at a time when the nurses themselves had a strong desire to broaden their role and enhance the status of their profession. A paper I published in the *Australian Journal of Advanced Nursing* (1987b) was positively received and I was invited to give addresses at maternal and child health conferences and in-service education courses where I was introduced as an 'honorary maternal and child health nurse'. These presentations were recorded on audio cassettes and videos so they could be used to reach nurses in rural areas. I also published papers in child welfare and mental health journals to reach other professional audiences and educate them about the central role of the maternal and child health nurse. During the decade following the study there was a marked growth in professional and public awareness and concern about post-natal depression and this also increased the profile of the study. [Mine] was one of the first studies on maternal depression and most [of those] that followed were large quantitative studies. Interestingly, these studies strongly supported the causal significance of the factors which I had identified the nurses using in assessing whether a mother was depressed (infant temperament and sleeping and eating problems; poor maternal family background; low level of support from partner and/or her own mother; and a number of situational stressors such as moving house,

illness, financial worries). The cumulative weight of the now large body of research carries consistent implications for policy and practice, and supports a broadened role for maternal and child health nurses. The transformation which had occurred in the maternal and child health service in Victoria, however, was threatened in the early 1990s by the election of the Kennett Government, which introduced policies which limited access to the service and narrowed the focus to one of 'paediatric surveillance'. Hence the campaign to protect the service and the mobilisation of mothers and their prams on the steps of Parliament. I think that the moral of this story for me is that researchers in the human services may well find themselves involved in giving a voice to those who have not been heard, and in joining a struggle for social justice.

Comments

As some of our inside stories illustrate, qualitative research is rarely a linear process and it often takes the researcher down unexpected pathways. The impact of the research may start very early on, and be part and parcel of the research itself, even in studies which are not thought of as 'action research'. Alternatively, the effects of the research may not register until some time after it has been completed and the impact will be largely determined by the receptivity of the prevailing climate.

Above all, our inside stories demonstrate that qualitative research in the human services is, as we have said before, not an end in itself but a means to an end. In that sense it is indeed 'mission-oriented research', and this book has drawn upon the experience of some particularly committed and enthusiastic missionaries!

The journey into the swampy lowlands of research, to use the phrase of Donald Schon with which we began the book, is more akin to a mystery tour than a trip which progresses along a set route from the start to the end. Because of this it is not possible to provide the aspiring qualitative researcher in the human services with a detailed map and a set of instructions which, if followed faithfully, will ensure that they get to their destination. Instead, we hope that through reporting the experiences of qualitative researchers who have undertaken prior expeditions, we have been able to provide a compass and some idea of the demands and delights of the diverse terrain which might be encountered on such journeys.

References

Adler, P. A. & Adler, P. 1987 *Membership Roles in Field Research*, Sage, Newbury Park, CA.

Alderson, P. (ed.) 1999 *Learning and Inclusion: The Cleves School Experience*, David Fulton, London.

Alkin, M. C. 1990 *Debates on Evaluation*, Sage, Newbury Park, CA.

Anderson, J. & Poole, M. 1998 *Assignment and Thesis Writing*, 3rd edn, John Wiley & Sons, Brisbane.

Backett, K. & Alexander, H. 1991 'Talking to young children about health: methods and findings' *Health Education Journal*, vol. 50, no. 1, pp. 34–8.

Basch, C. E. 1987 'Focus group interview: an underutilized research technique for improving theory and practice in health education' *Health Education Quarterly*, vol. 14, no. 4, pp. 411–48.

Bashford, L., Townsley, L. & Williams, C. 1995 'Parallel text: making research accessible to people with intellectual disabilities' *International Journal of Disability, Development and Education*, vol. 42, no. 3, pp. 211–20.

Becker, H. S. 1986 *Writing for Social Scientists*, University of Chicago Press, Chicago.

——1998 *Tricks of the Trade*, University of Chicago Press, Chicago.

Becker, H. S., Geer, B., Hughes, E. C. & Strauss, A. L. 1961 *Boys in White: Student Culture in Medical School*, University of Chicago Press, Chicago.

Becker, H. S., McCall, M. & Morris, L. 1989 'Theatres and communities: three scenes' *Social Problems*, vol. 36, pp. 93–116.

Beresford, B. 1997 *Personal Accounts: Involving Disabled Children in Research*, Social Policy Research Unit, Norwich.

Biklen, S. K. & Moseley, C. R. 1988 '"Are you retarded?" "No, I'm Catholic": qualitative methods in the study of people with severe handicaps' *Journal of the Association for Persons with Severe Handicaps*, vol. 13, no. 3, pp. 155–62.

Blalock, H. M. 1970 *An Introduction to Social Research*, Prentice-Hall, Englewood Cliffs, NJ.

Bogdan, R. C. & Biklen, S. K. 1992 *Qualitative Research for Education: An Introduction to Theory and Methods*, 2nd edn, Allyn & Bacon, Boston.

Booth, T. & Booth, W. 1994a *Parenting Under Pressure: Mothers and Fathers with Learning Difficulties*, Open University Press, Buckingham.

——1994b 'The use of depth interviewing with vulnerable subjects: lessons from a research study of parents with learning difficulties' *Social Science and Medicine*, vol. 39, no. 3, pp. 415–24.

——1996 'Sounds of silence: narrative research with inarticulate subjects' *Disability and Society*, vol. 11, no. 1, pp. 55–69.

——1998 *Growing Up With Parents Who Have Learning Difficulties*, Routledge, London.

Booth, W. 1998 'Doing research with lonely people' *British Journal of Learning Difficulties*, vol. 26, no. 4, pp. 132–4.

Borland, M., Laybourn, A., Hill, M. & Brown, J. 1998 *Middle Childhood: The Perspectives of Children and Parents*, Jessica Kingsley, London.

Bostwick, G. & Kyte, N. 1981 'Measurement' in R. Grinnell (ed.) *Social Work Research and Evaluation*, F. E. Peacock & Sons, Itasca, Il.

Brannen, J. & O'Brien, M. 1995 'Childhood and the sociological gaze: paradigms and paradoxes' *Sociology*, vol. 29, no. 4, pp. 729–37.

Brenner, M., Brown, J. & Canter, D. 1985 'Introduction' in M. Brenner, J. Brown, J. & D. Canter (eds) *The Research Interview: Uses and Approaches*, Academic Press, London, pp. 1–8.

Bruner, E. M. 1986 'Ethnography as narrative' in V. W. Turner & E. M. Bruner (eds) *The Anthropology of Experience*, University of Illinois Press, Chicago, pp. 139–55.

Bryman, A. 1988 *Quality and Quantity in Social Research*, Unwin Hyman, London.

——1992 'Quantitative and qualitative research: further reflections on their integration' in J. Brannen (ed.) *Mixing Methods: Qualitative and Quantitative Research,* Avebury, Aldershot, pp. 57–78.

Burgess, R. G. 1984 *In the Field: An Introduction to Field Research,* George Allen & Unwin, London.

Burnside 2000 *Research Code of Ethics,* Burnside, North Parramatta.

Butler, I. & Williamson, H. 1994 *Children Speak: Children, Trauma and Social Work,* Longman, Harlow.

Carey, S. 1985 *Conceptual Change in Childhood,* Massachusetts Institute of Technology Press, Cambridge, MA.

Coleman, A. 1997 'Empty streets: current policy relating to long-term homelessness' in P. Saunders & T. Eardley (eds) *States, Markets and Communities: Remapping the Boundaries Volume 1,* Social Policy Research Centre, Sydney, pp. 59–71.

——2001 'Five star motels: spaces, places and homelessness in Fortitude Valley' unpublished PhD Dissertation, The University of Queensland.

Collaizzi, P. F. 1978 'Psychological research as the phenomenologist views it' in R. S. Valle & M. King (eds) *Existential-phenomenological Alternatives for Psychology,* Oxford University Press, New York, pp. 48–71.

Cook, T. D. & Reichardt, C. S. 1979 *Qualitative and Quantitative Methods in Evaluation Research,* Sage, Beverley Hills, CA.

Commonwealth Department of Human Services and Health 1995 *Ethical Research and Ethics Committee Review of Social and Behavioral Research Proposals,* AGPS, Canberra.

Corsaro, W. A. 1985 *Friendship and Peer Culture in the Early Years,* Ablex, Norwood, NJ.

Cousins, J. B. & Leithwood, K. A. 1986 'Current empirical research on evaluation utilization' *Review of Educational Research,* vol. 56, no. 3, pp. 331–64.

Dalton, M. 1959 *Men Who Manage,* Wiley, New York.

Darlington, Y. 1993 'The experience of childhood sexual abuse: perspectives of adult women who were sexually abused in childhood' unpublished PhD Dissertation, The University of Queensland.

——1996 *Moving On: Women's Experiences of Childhood Sexual Abuse and Beyond,* The Federation Press, Sydney.

Darlington, Y. & Bland, R. 1999 'Strategies for encouraging and maintaining hope among people living with serious mental illness' *Australian Social Work,* vol. 52, no. 3, pp. 17–23.

References

Darlington, Y., Osmond, J. & Peile, C. 2002 'Child welfare workers' use of theory in working with physical child abuse: implications for professional supervision' *Families in Society*, in press.

Deetz, S. 1985 'Ethical considerations in cultural research in organizations' P. Frost, L. Moore, M. Louis, C. Lundberg & J. Martin (eds) *Organizational Culture*, Sage, Beverly Hills, pp. 253–69.

Dey, I. 1993 *Qualitative Data Analysis: A User-Friendly Guide for Social Scientists*, Routledge, London.

Donaldson, M. 1978 *Children's Minds*, Fontana/Collins, Glasgow.

Fielding, N. G. & Lee, R. M. 1998 *Computer Analysis and Qualitative Research*, Sage, London.

Filstead, W. J. 1979 'Qualitative methods: a needed perspective in evaluation research' in T. D. Cook & C. S. Reichardt (eds) *Qualitative and Quantitative Methods in Evaluation Research*, Sage, Beverly Hills, CA, pp. 33–48.

Finch, J. 1984 '"It's great to have someone to talk to": the ethics and politics of interviewing women' in C. Bell & H. Roberts (eds) *Social Researching: Politics, Problems and Practice*, Routledge & Kegan Paul, London, pp. 70–87.

Fine, G. A. & Sandstrom, K. L. 1988 *Knowing Children: Participant Observation with Minors*, Sage, Newbury Park, CA.

Fraser, M. & Leavitt, S. 1990 'Creating social change: "mission"-oriented research and entrepreneurship' in J. Whittaker, J. Kinney, M. Tracy & C. Booth (eds) *Reaching High Risk Families*, Aldine, New York, pp. 165–78.

Gans, H. J. 1982 'The participant observer as a human being: observations on the personal aspects of fieldwork' in R. G. Burgess (ed.) *Field Research: A Sourcebook and Field Manual*, George Allen & Unwin, London, pp. 53–61.

Gee, J. P. 1999 *An Introduction to Discourse Analysis: Theory and Method*, Routledge, London.

Glaser, B. G. & Strauss, A. L. 1967 *The Discovery of Grounded Theory*, Aldine, New York.

Gold, R. L. 1958 'Roles in sociological field observation' *Social Forces*, vol. 36, pp. 217–23.

Goode, D. A. 1986 'Kids, culture and innocents' *Human Studies*, vol. 9, pp. 83–106.

Grbich, C. 1999 *Qualitative Research in Health: An Introduction*, Allen & Unwin, Sydney.

Greene, J. C., Caracelli, V. J. & Graham, W. F. 1989 'Toward a conceptual framework for mixed-method evaluation designs' *Educational Evaluation and Policy Analysis*, vol. 11, no. 3, pp. 255–74.

Guba, E. G. 1985 'The context of emergent paradigm research' in Y. S. Lincoln (ed.) *Organizational Theory and Inquiry: The Paradigm Revolution*, Sage, Beverly Hills, CA, pp. 79–104.

Guba, E. G. & Lincoln, Y. S. 1989 *Fourth Generation Evaluation*, Sage, Newbury Park, CA.

Hammersley, M. & Atkinson, P. 1995 *Ethnography: Principles in Practice*, 2nd edn, Routledge, London.

Harding, S. 1986 *The Science Question in Feminism*, Cornell University Press, Ithaca, NJ.

Health Education Board for Scotland 1997 *Messages from Children*, Health Education Board for Scotland, Edinburgh.

Hendricks, M. & Papagiannis, M. 1990 'Do's and don'ts for effective recommendations' *Evaluation Practice*, vol. 11, no. 2, pp. 121–5.

Hersen, M. & Barlow, D. 1976 *Single Case Experimental Designs*, Pergamon Press, Elmsford, NY.

Hill, M., Laybourn, A. & Borland, M. 1996 'Engaging with primary-aged children about their emotions and well-being: methodological considerations' *Children and Society*, vol. 10, no. 2, pp. 129–44.

Holstein, J. A. & Gubrium, J. F. 1994 'Phenomenology, ethno-methodology and interpretive practice' in N. K. Denzin & Y. S. Lincoln (eds) *Handbook of Qualitative Research*, Sage, Thousand Oaks, CA, pp. 262–72.

——1995 *The Active Interview*, Sage, Thousand Oaks, CA.

——1997 'Active interviewing' in D. Silverman (ed.) *Qualitative Research: Theory, Method and Practice*, Sage, London, pp. 113–29.

Hood, S., Kelley, P. & Mayall, B. 1996 'Children as research subjects: a risky enterprise' *Children and Society*, vol. 10, no. 2, pp. 117–28.

Hoppe, M. J., Wells, E. A., Morrison, D. M., Gillmore, M. R. & Wilsdon, A. 1995 'Using focus groups to discuss sensitive topics with children' *Evaluation Review*, vol. 19, no. 1, pp. 102–14.

Hyde, C. 1994 'Reflections on a journey: a research story' in C. K. Riessman (ed.) *Qualitative Studies in Social Work Research*, Sage, Thousand Oaks, CA, pp. 169–89.

Imle, M. A. & Atwood, J. R. 1988 'Retaining qualitative validity while gaining quantitative reliability and validity: development of the Transition to Parenthood Concerns scale' *Advances in Nursing Science*, vol. 11, no. 1, pp. 61–75.

Johnson, K. & Scott, D. 1997 'Confessional tales: an exploration of the self and other in two ethnographies' *Australian Journal of Social Research*, vol. 4, no. 1, pp. 27–48.

Johnson, J. M. 1975 *Doing Field Research*, The Free Press, New York.

Keil, F. C. 1989 *Concepts, Kinds and Cognitive Development*, Massachusetts Institute of Technology Press, Cambridge, MA.

Kelly, L. 1999 *Domestic Violence Matters: An Evaluation of a Development Project*, Home Office, London.

Kidder, L. H. & Fine, M. 1987 'Qualitative and quantitative methods: when stories converge' in M. M. Mark & R. L. Shotland (eds) *Multiple Methods in Program Evaluation: New Directions for Program Evaluation 35*, Jossey-Bass, San Francisco, pp. 57–75.

Kleinman, A. 1988 *The Illness Narratives: Suffering, Healing and the Human Condition*, Basic Books, New York.

Koocher, G. & Keith-Spiegel, P. 1994 'Scientific issues in psychosocial and educational research with children' in M. Grodin & L. Glantz (eds) *Children as Research Subjects: Science, Ethics and Law*, Oxford University Press, New York, pp. 47–80.

Krahn, G. L., Hohn, M. F. & Kime, C. 1995 'Incorporating qualitative approaches into clinical child psychology research' *Journal of Clinical Child Psychology*, vol. 24, no. 2, pp. 204–13.

Langness, L. L. & Frank, G. 1981 *Lives: An Anthropological Approach to Biography*, Chandler & Sharp, Novato, CA.

Laurie, H. 1992 'Multiple methods in the study of household resource allocation' in J. Brannen (ed.) *Mixing Methods: Qualitative and Quantitative Research*, Avebury, Aldershot, pp. 145–68.

Lewins, F. 1993 *Writing a Thesis*, 4th edn, Faculty of Arts, Australian National University, Canberra.

Liebow, E. 1967 *Tally's Corner*, Little, Brown, Boston.

——1993 *Tell Them Who I Am: The Lives of Homeless Women*, Penguin, New York.

Lofland, J. & Lofland, L. H. 1995 *Analyzing Social Settings: A Guide to Qualitative Observation and Analysis*, 3rd edn, Wadsworth, Belmont.

Mandell, N. 1988 'The least-adult role in studying children' *Journal of Contemporary Ethnography*, vol. 16, no. 4, pp. 433–67.

Marcus, G. 1994 'What comes (just) after post? The case of ethnography' in N. Denzin & Y. Lincoln (eds) *Handbook of Qualitative Research*, Sage, Thousand Oaks, CA, pp. 563–74.

Mariampolski, H. 1989 'Focus groups on sensitive topics: how to get subjects to open up and feel good about telling the truth' *Applied Marketing Research*, vol. 29, no. 1, pp. 6–11.

Mark, M. M. & Shotland, R. L. (eds) 1987 *Multiple Methods in Program Evaluation: New Directions for Program Evaluation 35,* Jossey-Bass, San Francisco.

Mason, J. 1996 *Qualitative Researching,* Sage, London.

Mates, D. & Allison, K. R. 1992 'Sources of stress and coping responses of high school students' *Adolescence,* vol. 27, no. 106, pp. 461–74.

Matocha, L. K. 1992 'Case study interviews: caring for persons with AIDS' in J. F. Gilgun, K. Daly & G. Handel (eds) *Qualitative Methods in Family Research,* Sage, Newbury Park, CA, pp. 66–84.

Mayall, B. 1999 'Children and childhood' in S. Hood, B. Mayall & S. Oliver (eds) *Critical Issues in Social Research: Power and Prejudice,* Open University Press, Buckingham, pp. 10–24.

McAuliffe, D. & Coleman, A. 1999 'Damned if we do and damned if we don't: exposing ethical tensions in field research' *Australian Social Work,* vol. 52, no. 4, pp. 25–31.

McCall, M. M., Becker, H. S. & Meshejian, P. 1990 'Performance science' *Social Problems,* vol. 37, no. 1, pp. 117–32.

McDonald, C. 1996 'Institutionalised organisations? A study of nonprofit human service organisations' unpublished PhD Dissertation, The University of Queensland.

——1997 'Government, funded nonprofits and accountability' *Nonprofit Management and Leadership,* vol. 8, pp. 51–64.

——1999 'Internal control and accountability in nonprofit human service organisations' *Australian Journal of Public Administration,* vol. 58, no. 1, pp. 11–22.

Melton, G. B. & Flood, M. F. 1994 'Research policy and child maltreatment: developing the scientific foundation for effective protection of children' *Child Abuse and Neglect,* vol. 18 (Supplement 1), no. 1, pp. 1–28.

Miles, M. B. & Huberman, A. M. 1994 *Qualitative Data Analysis: An Expanded Sourcebook,* 2nd edn, Sage, Thousand Oaks, CA.

Miller, J. & Glassner, B. 1997 'The "inside" and the "outside": finding realities in interviews' in D. Silverman (ed.) *Qualitative Research: Theory, Method and Practice,* Sage, London, pp. 99–112.

Miller, W. and Crabtree, B. 1992 'Primary care research: a multi-methods typology and qualitative road map' in B. Crabtree & W. Miller (eds) *Doing Qualitative Research: Research Methods for Primary Care,* vol. 3, Sage, Newbury Park, CA, pp. 3–28.

Minichiello, V., Aroni, R., Timewell, E. & Alexander, L. 1990 *In-depth Interviewing: Researching People,* Longman Cheshire, Melbourne.

——1995 *In-depth Interviewing: Principles, Techniques, Analysis*, 2nd edn, Longman, Melbourne.

Minkes, J., Robinson, C. & Weston, C. 1994 'Consulting the children: interviews with children using residential respite care services' *Disability and Society*, vol. 9, no. 1, pp. 47–57.

Moran-Ellis, J. 1996 'Close to home: the experience of researching child sexual abuse' in M. Hester, L. Kelly & J. Radford (eds) *Women, Violence and Male Power: Feminist Activism, Research and Practice*, Open University Press, Buckingham, pp. 176–87.

Morgan, D. L. 1997 *Focus Groups as Qualitative Research*, 2nd edn, Sage, Newbury Park, CA.

Morse, J. M. 1994 'Designing funded qualitative research' in N. K. Denzin & Y. S. Lincoln (eds) *Handbook of Qualitative Research*, Sage, Thousand Oaks, CA, pp. 220–35.

Munford, R., Sanders, J., Tisdall, M., Jack, A., Mulder, J. & Spoonley, P. 1996 *Working Successfully with Families: Stage 1*, Barnardos New Zealand, Wellington.

Munford, R., Sanders, J., Tisdall, M., Henare, A., Livingstone, K. & Spoonley, P. 1998 *Working Successfully with Families: Stage 2*, Barnardos New Zealand, Wellington.

Munford, R. & Sanders, J. 1999 *Supporting Families*, Dunmore Press, Palmerston North, NZ.

——2000a 'Ethical issues in qualitative research with families' in M. Tollich (ed.) *Ethical Issues for Qualitative Research*, Pearson Education, Longman, Auckland, pp. 99–112.

——2000b 'Through the eyes of the actors: three challenges for qualitative research with families' *International Journal of Qualitative Health Research*, vol. 10, no. 6, pp. 841–53.

Murphy, E. 1985 *You Can Write: A Do-it-yourself Manual*, Longman Cheshire, Melbourne.

National Health and Medical Research Council 1995 *Ethics Aspects of Qualitative Methods in Health Research: An Information Paper for Institutional Ethics Committees*, Commonwealth Department of Health and Family Services, Australian Government Publishing Service, Canberra.

1999 *National Statement on Ethical Conduct in Research Involving Humans*, Commonwealth Department of Health and Family Services, Australian Government Publishing Service, Canberra.

Oakley, A. 1981 'Interviewing women: a contradiction in terms' in H. Roberts (ed.) *Doing Feminist Research*, Routledge & Kegan Paul, London, pp. 30–61.

——'People's ways of knowing: gender and methodology' in S. Hood, B. Mayall & S. Oliver (eds) *Critical Issues in Social Research: Power and Prejudice*, Open University Press, Buckingham, pp. 154–70.

Owen, J. M. & Rogers, P. J. 1999 *Program Evaluation: Forms and Approaches*, 2nd edn, Allen & Unwin, Sydney.

Padgett, D. K. 1998 *Qualitative Methods in Social Work: Challenges and Rewards*, Sage, Thousand Oaks, CA.

Paget, M. A. 1990 'Performing the text' *Journal of Contemporary Ethnography*, vol. 19, no. 1, pp. 136–55.

Patton, M. 1988 'The future of evaluation' *Evaluation Practice*, vol. 9, no. 4, pp. 90–3.

——1990 *Qualitative Evaluation and Research Methods*, Sage, Newbury Park, CA.

Patton, M. Q. 1997 *Utilization-focused Evaluation: The New Century Text*, 3rd edn, Sage, Thousand Oaks, CA.

Pe-Pua, R. 1996 *We're Just Like Other Kids: Street-frequenting Youth of Non-English-speaking Background*, Bureau of Immigration, Multicultural and Population Research, Australian Government Publishing Service, Canberra.

Pirkis, J. & Gardner, H. 1998 'Writing for publication' *Australian Journal of Public Health—Interchange*, vol. 4, no. 2, pp. 71–6.

Polkinghorne, D. E. 1989 'Phenomenological research methods' in R. S. Valle & S. Halling (eds) *Existential–Phenomenological Perspectives in Psychology*, Plenum Press, New York, pp. 41–60.

Psathas, G. 1995 *Conversation Analysis: The Study of Talk-in-interaction*, Sage, Thousand Oaks, CA.

Ramos, M., 1989 'Some ethical implications of qualitative research' *Research in Nursing and Health*, 12, pp. 57–63.

Reicher, S. & Emler, N. 1986 'Managing reputations in adolescence: the pursuit of delinquent and non-delinquent identities' in H. Beloff (ed.) *Getting into Life* , Methuen, London, pp. 13–42.

Rein, M. & White, S. 1981 'Knowledge for practice' *Social Service Review*, vol. 55, no. 1, pp. 1–41.

Ribbens, J. 1989 'Interviewing—an "unnatural situation"?' *Women's Studies International Forum*, vol. 12, no. 6, pp. 579–92.

Richardson, L. 1985 *The New Other Woman: Contemporary Single Women in Affairs with Married Men*, Free Press, New York.

——1986 'Another world' *Psychology Today*, vol. 20, no. 2, pp. 22–7.

——1988 'Secrecy and status: the social construction of forbidden relationships' *American Sociological Review*, vol. 53, no. 2, pp. 209–20.

——1990 *Writing Strategies: Reaching Diverse Audiences*, Sage, Newbury Park, CA.

Riessman, C. K. 1993 *Narrative Analysis*, Sage, Newbury Park, CA.

Rist, R. C. 1977 'On the relations among educational research paradigms: from disdain to detente' *Anthropology and Education Quarterly*, vol. 8, no. 1, pp. 42–9.

Rosenhan, D. L. 1973 'On being sane in insane places' *Science*, vol. 179, pp. 250–8.

Rountree, K. & Laing, T. 1996 *Writing by Degrees: A Practical Guide to Writing Theses and Research Papers*, Addison Wesley Longman, Auckland.

Sanders, J., Munford, R. & Richards-Ward, L. 1999 *Working Successfully with Families: Stage 3*, Barnardos New Zealand, Wellington.

Schon, D. A. 1983 *The Reflective Practitioner: How Professionals Think in Action*, Temple Smith, London.

Scott, D. 1987a 'Primary intervention in maternal depression' unpublished Master of Social Work Thesis, University of Melbourne.

——1987b 'Maternal and child health nurse role in post-partum depression' *Australian Journal of Advanced Nursing*, vol. 5, no. 1, pp. 28–37.

——1989 'Meaning construction and social work practice' *Social Service Review*, vol. 63, pp. 39–51.

——1990 'Practice wisdom: the neglected source of practice research', *Social Work*, vol. 35, no. 6, pp. 564–8.

——1992 'Early identification of maternal depression as a strategy in the prevention of child abuse' *Child Abuse and Neglect*, vol. 16, pp. 345–58.

——1995 'Child protection assessment: an ecological perspective' unpublished PhD Dissertation, School of Social Work, University of Melbourne.

Scott, R.W. 1969 'Field methods in the study of organizations' in A. Etzioni (ed.) *A Sociological Reader on Complex Organizations*, Holt, Rinehart & Winston Inc., New York, pp. 558–76.

Seidel, J. 1998 *The Ethnograph v5.0*, Qualis Research Associates, Thousand Oaks, CA.

Siegert, M. T. 1986 'Adult elicited child behavior: the paradox of measuring social competence through interviewing' in J. Cook-Gumperz, W. A. Corsaro & J. Streeck (eds) *Children's Worlds and Children's Language*, Mouton de Gruyter, Berlin, pp. 359–76.

Singh, N. N., Curtis, W. J., Wechsler, H. A., Ellis, C. R. & Cohen, R. 1997 'Family friendliness of community-based services for children and adolescents with emotional and behavioral disorders and their families: an observational study' *Journal of Emotional and Behavioral Disorders*, vol. 5, no. 2, pp. 82–92.

Smith, J. K. & Heshusius, L. 1986 'Closing down the conversation: the end of the quantitative–qualitative debate among educational inquirers' *Educational Researcher*, vol. 15, no. 1, pp. 4–12.

Spradley, J. P. 1980 *Participant Observation*, Holt, Rinehart & Winston, New York.

Stacey, J. 1988 'Can there be a feminist ethnography?' *Women's Studies International Forum*, vol. 11, no. 1, pp. 21–7.

Stanley, L. & Wise, S. 1983 *Breaking Out: Feminist Consciousness and Feminist Research*, Routledge & Kegan Paul, London.

Steward, M. S., Bussey, K., Goodman, G. S. & Saywitz, K. J. 1993 'Implications of developmental research for interviewing children' *Child Abuse and Neglect*, vol. 17, pp. 25–37.

Strauss, A. 1987 *Qualitative Analysis for Social Scientists*, Cambridge University Press, Cambridge.

Strauss, A. L. & Corbin, J. 1990 *Basics of Qualitative Research: Techniques and Procedures for Developing Grounded Theory*, Sage, Thousand Oaks, CA.

Strauss, A. L. & Corbin, J. 1998 *Basics of Qualitative Research: Grounded Theory Procedures and Techniques*, 2nd edn, Sage, Thousand Oaks, CA.

Strunk, W. & White, E. B. 2000 *The Elements of Style*, 4th edn, Macmillan, New York.

Tammivaara, J. & Enright, D. S. 1986 'On eliciting information: dialogues with child informants' *Anthropology and Education Quarterly*, vol. 17, no. 1, pp. 218–38.

Taylor, S. J. & Bogdan, R. 1998 *Introduction to Qualitative Research Methods*, 3rd edn, John Wiley & Son, New York.

Tesch, R. 1990 *Qualitative Research: Analysis Types and Software Tools*, The Falmer Press, New York.

Thomas, C., Beckford, V., Lowe, N. & Murch, M. 1999 *Adopted Children Speaking*, British Agencies for Adoption and Fostering, London.

Thomas, E. J. 1978 'Generating innovation in social work: the paradigm of developmental research' *Journal of Social Service Research*, 2, pp. 95–115.

Tilse, C. 1994 'Long term marriage and long term care' *Australian Journal on Ageing*, vol. 13, no. 4, pp. 172–4.

——1996 'The long goodbye: the experience of placing and visiting a long term partner in a nursing home' unpublished PhD Dissertation, The University of Queensland.

——1997a 'Family advocacy roles and highly dependent residents in nursing homes' *Australian Journal on Ageing*, vol. 16, no. 1, pp. 20–3.

——1997b 'Resources, rights and relationships: family participation in residential care' in P. Saunders & T. Eardley (eds) *States, Markets and Communities: Remapping the Boundaries Volume 2*, Social Policy Research Centre, Sydney, pp. 121–30.

Tomm, K. 1988 'Interventive interviewing: part III. Intending to ask lineal, circular, strategic or reflexive questions?' *Family Process*, vol. 27, no. 1, pp. 1–15.

Trickett, P. K. 1993 'Maladaptive development of school-aged, physically abused children: relationships with the child-rearing context' *Journal of Family Psychology*, vol. 7, pp. 134–47.

Trinder, L., Beek, M. & Connolly, J. 2001 *The Contact Project First Year: Interim Report for the Advisory Committee*, University of East Anglia, Norwich.

United Nations Centre for Human Rights 1989 *Convention on the Rights of the Child*, United Nations, Geneva.

van Maanen, J. 1988 *Tales of the Field: On Writing Ethnography*, University of Chicago Press, Chicago.

Wade, B. & Moore, M. 1993 *Experiencing Special Education: What Young People with Special Education Needs Can Tell Us*, Open University Press, Buckingham.

Walker, R. 1985 'An introduction to applied qualitative research' in R. Walker (ed.) *Applied Qualitative Research*, Gower, Aldershot, Hants, pp. 3–26.

Ward, L. 1997 *Seen and Heard: Involving Disabled Children and Young People in Research and Development Projects*, Joseph Rowntree Foundation, York.

Ward, L. & Simons, K. 1998 'Practising partnership: involving people with learning difficulties in research' *British Journal of Learning Difficulties*, vol. 26, no. 4, pp. 128–31.

Weiss, C. H. 1990 'Evaluation for decisions: Is anybody there? Does anybody care?' in M. C. Alkin (ed.) *Debates on Evaluation*, Sage, Newbury Park, CA, pp. 171–84.

Weiss, C. H. & Bucuvalas, M. J. 1980 *Social Science Research and Decision-Making*, Columbia University Press, New York.

Wertz, F. J. & van Zuuren, F. J. 1987 'Qualitative research: educational considerations' in F. J. Van Zuuren, F. J. Wertz & B. Mook (eds) *Advances in Qualitative Psychology: Themes and Variations*, Swets North America, Berwyn, PA, pp. 3–23.

Wilkinson, M. 1993 'Children's rights: debates and dilemmas' in J. Mason (ed.) *Child Welfare Policy: Critical Australian Perspectives*, Hale & Iremonger, Sydney, pp. 143–56.

Williams, L. F. & Hopps, J. G. 1988 'On the nature of professional communication: publication for practitioners' *Social Work*, vol. 33, no. 5, pp. 453–9.

Wolcott, H. F. 1990 *Writing Up Qualitative Research*, Sage, Newbury Park, CA.

Woods, P. 1985 'New songs played skilfully: creativity and technique in writing up qualitative research' in R. G. Burgess (ed.) *Issues in Educational Research: Qualitative Methods*, The Falmer Press, London, pp. 86–106.

Yuen-Tsang, A. W. K. 1997 *Towards a Chinese Conception of Social Support: A Study on the Social Support Networks of Chinese Working Mothers in Beijing*, Ashgate, Aldershot.

Index

Page numbers in italics refer to interviews